INTERMITTENT FASTING FOR WOMEN

The Ultimate Guide and Step by Step Tutorial for Fast Weight Loss, Autophagy Process and Easy Solutions to Improve the Quality of Life

David S. Kingston

INTRODUCTION

"Fasting" is the total or partial abstention of food and drink at a specific time.

"Intermittent" means that this fasting is interrupted in a regularly controlled manner (if not intermittent, it will remain indefinitely over time and sooner or later we will die)

Intermittent fasting is a pattern of meals (not meals) that alternates between full and partial abstentions of meals and / or drinks on a regular and controlled basis.

Therefore intermittent fasting does not control what you eat or drink, but it controls when you do it. Every day we fast naturally during the period from dinner to breakfast (hence terms such as "fasting glucose" taken in some of the regular health checks).

But other times of fasting are also not new to humans: the ability to survive and develop properly functioning mechanisms and adaptations during periods of food shortage was an important element of human evolutionary history

If you have tried other diets and feel that they are too difficult to follow, expensive or that take a long time, then you are not alone!

If you are a busy person and do not have time to follow a fad diet, then intermittent fasting is the perfect diet for you!

It does not require going to the gym or buying accessories for training.

You can eat whatever you want, according to your own time.

You do not need to count calories or consume specific foods.

And best of all, it's free!

Fasting is much easier than you imagine. You can continue eating your favorite foods, feeling and looking much better.

CHAPTER ONE

ORIGIN OF INTERMITTENT FASTING

Fasting is not a new concept. For centuries, people have temporarily restricted food intake for religious reasons. Over the past few years, intermittent fasting has attracted attention for its incredible impact on illness and aging when eating nothing for 16 to 48 hours (or more).

Fasting is one of the topics that arouse most interest in regard to nutrition and health. Let's see why: what is fasting, what effects it has on the body and how to do it.

Fasting is a stop in food intake that allows a global set-up of the body.

Debugging and fasting are natural practices , common to many species: those who have cats and dogs will have seen that they stop eating and purge when they have been intoxicated, most animals stop eating while they heal from fractures or wounds, Migratory birds stop eating for long periods of time and bears fast during hibernation.

The human being, too, the human being is adapted to periods of scarcity and, naturally, also fasts when he is sick.

Purifying diets and fasting have been present throughout the history of mankind. There are data on these practices in Babylon, China, India, Greece, Palestine, Persia, Rome. Fasting was practiced and recommended by doctors of ancient Hippocrates or Galen for the treatment and prevention of diseases. It was also the practice of the great thinkers Aristotle, Plato and Socrates and from religious teachers like Moses, Buddha, Jesus Christ and Muhammad.

Fasting is used for the preparation of religious celebrations. It is usual practice of yogis. The Lent of Christians prepares for Easter, a period of purification of body and soul; and it is inspired by one of the most famous fasts in history: the 40-day period that Jesus Christ spent in the desert without taking food or drink. The Ramadan of Muslims is a period of restriction of food and drink during the hours of the sun to enhance internalization and detach from the ego.

In the twentieth century, therapeutic fasting reappeared in the West (USA and Europe) and its therapeutic indications were rescued. Today it is one of the most current issues related to food and health

WHAT IS FASTING

Fasting is the action of fasting or not eating food. A prolonged fast causes a lack of nutrients and energy sources that cause changes in the structure and function of the organs and even death.

Autophagy has attracted a great deal of interest among researchers since its discovery in the 1960s. Fasting has been used in traditional medicine since time immemorial. Now, we understand better why tradition teaches that when the body is released from the work of digestion, it uses its energy to eliminate waste and repair itself.

WHAT IS INTERMITTENT FASTING

This type of diet consists of alternating periods of fasting shorter or longer and periods of food intake. Much more flexible and accessible than strict fasting that allows no food intake, intermittent fasting provides the same health benefits. There are different ways to do intermittent fasting: partial fasting, 5: 2, fasting, etc.

Current dietary trends include intermittent fasting. More than a diet, this new way of eating would have many health benefits. Fasting to lose weight would have even become the new slimming secret. In this article, discover the real benefits of fasting and how to practice it with a typical fasting menu day.

FASTING PROMOTES A HEALTHIER OLD AGE

Until relatively recently, most human groups practiced fasting regularly. Fasting has been practiced, historically, for religious, political, spiritual, and environmental or health reasons; In prehistory, during the long-term hunting-gathering system, our ancestors went from extensive periods of high caloric restriction or fasting to feasts in times of bonanza.

Human evolution was marked by this cycle of fasting and feasts. Long before, at the beginning of eukaryotic life, the cells implemented a catabolic process known as autophagy in response to the same cycle of abundance and lack or absence of nutrients in the environment: Autophagy.

Autophagy is, then, an adaptation against starvation: a regulated mechanism of destruction of damaged or unnecessary parts of the cells; aberrant organelles and other cellular components are sequestered, degraded and recycled, in addition to maintaining optimal energy levels in the cell. Fasting (particularly after 24 hours) causes the process of autophagy and autophagy covers the body's energy needs while promoting cell regeneration.

Now, although autophagy was identified as a biological process in the 1960s, today its functioning at the molecular level is still poorly understood. Autophagy studies have multiplied in the last 15 years and their results are surprising: it is essential for homeostasis; its absence promotes the accumulation of damaged cells; lack of autophagy is also a dominant factor in the appearance of age-related disorders, such as osteoatritis; it is linked to the appearance and progression of different types of cancer, as well as to the suppression of tumors; produces longevity in certain organisms; It is essential for neuronal survival and the efficacy of fasting and autophagy therapies to treat Parkinson's and Alzheimers diseases is currently being analyzed.

It is worth clarifying that autophagy is not a panacea, it is only a biological regulatory process whose functions we have annulled with the introduction of Western food culture; that is, never go hungry and whenever you eat, eat a feast.

Here we present just one of the most recent studies on autophagy in mammals: Through a single mutation induced in the Becn-1 gene (becline 1), researchers from the University of the Northwest, in Chicago, promoted high levels of autophagy in laboratory mice Mice with the mutation in this gene, which has a critical function in autophagy and cell death, showed greater longevity than normal mice, as well as a delay in the degeneration of renal and cardiac functions.

This shows that increasing autophagy is an effective method to promote healthier aging," said Congcong He, co-author of the study, "disorders related to an advanced age, such as Alzheimers, reduce the well-being of the patient, his family and the whole society. " Autophagy in mammals, summarizing,

WHY SHOULD I DO INTERMITTENT FASTING

Intermittent fasting specifically offers the added advantage of allowing progressive entry to fasting for those who want to start in this world. It is also an interesting use supplement for veterans who practice prolonged fasting and do not want to limit their practice only to the occasions reserved for long-term fasting.

Unlike long-term fasting, in which the way to enter and leave the fasting is important , in intermittent fasting this does not have great relevance, since the objective is to extend the interval between meals as much as possible and there are no changes Metabolic as deep as when we spend days without eating any food.

So, to make intermittent fasting, you simply have to continue with the healthy nutritional guidelines that work for you, lengthening the hours you spend fasting and compressing the time window in which you include your meals.

The truth is that there are a number of advantages of intermittent fasting from which we can benefit:

First, scientific studies have shown that intermittent fasting makes us less resistant to insulin.
Other studies suggest that people who fast have more energy, better cognition and memory, as well as increased production of the so-called neuro-trophic growth factor (a protein that promotes the growth and protection of neurons).

A study alleges not eating for a period of time puts cells in a state of less stress, making them better able to fend for themselves in other stress situations.

Other studies that analyzed people participating in Ramadan claimed that intermittent fasting could improve our immunity, decrease the risk of diabetes and improve our heart health.

FASTING AND DETOXIFICATION

In addition to stopping any possibility of ingesting toxins, fasting would have a detoxifying action, mainly by activating autophagy. This detoxification is more powerful than with a simple hypotoxic diet. It is exercised inside our cells.

This is very interesting because the majority of the techniques of detoxification aim rather at the elimination of the toxins contained in the blood or in the environment where our cells bathe (and who nourishes them).

These techniques evacuate the toxins by the elimination organs (liver, kidney, colon). Autophagy cleans and restores the inside of the cells at the same time .

Fasting can be done for different reasons:

Fasting to lose weight. There is a belief that to lose weight you must fast. However, it can cause serious health problems and is associated with eating disorders such as anorexia. There are other methods of slimming more recommended and that do not contemplate fasting.

Spiritual fast . It is done for religious or spiritual reasons. Some examples of fasting associated with religious beliefs are fasting during Yon Kippur and fasting during the month of Ramadan.

Fasting to perform a blood test . Certain types of medical tests are performed 'on an empty stomach'. It is due to physiological reasons, since it is intended to obtain a sample 'under normal conditions' and some parameters change after eating food, for example, cholesterol or transaminases. It is also because the reference values are standardized based on a healthy and fasting population analysis.

Fasting days

In Catholic doctrine , fasting is considered to make only one strong meal a day and two small meals that do not exceed the main meal altogether. This must be done on Ash Wednesday and Good Friday. The withdrawal is not eating red meat. Withdrawal days are considered every Friday and Ash Wednesday. There are some dispensations and commutations established in Canon Law. These forms of penance may vary as they are established by the Episcopal Conference of each country.

Breakfast

The word breakfast in its origin means the opposite of 'fasting'. It is commonly applied to food that is done at the beginning of the day and that ends the period of fasting during sleeping hours.

Other reasons for fasting

Fasting, it is occasions, can also be used as a form of protest, known as a hunger strike. In some natural medicine streams, fasting is used to combat some diseases.

WHAT HAPPENS WHEN WE STOP FEEDING

Our organization is very familiar with the adaptation process that needs to be followed. For millions of years it has been part of our genetic heritage. Everything is set up naturally, according to a procedure now well known:

During the first thirty hours, the human body functions on immediately available reserves, drawing on muscle and liver glycogen stores . The production of glucose is provided by glycogenesis, which is what usually allows us to have a physical activity without having to feed us continuously.

Beyond this period, the glycogen reserves being

exhausted, a double metabolic flip-flop gradually sets in place. On the one hand the gluconeogenesis that will produce sugar from the proteins, and on the other hand the lipolysis, degradation of the fats which constitute our reserves in the long term. T

he ones we never use, since for most of us the diet is repeated two to three times a day since birth. Then, very quickly (most often within a dozen hours), the human body will give priority to the use of fat.

Indeed the consumption of proteins is mainly at the expense of muscle mass, but the heart is a muscle. By transforming body fat into ketone bodies, the metabolism naturally exploits a source of energy that quickly becomes dominant as long as no external energy supply occurs.

Precise measurements of this adaptation to the absence of food intake confirm that there are variations among species, but that they always occur, according to a relatively standardized progression.

HOW TO FAST

First, understand that there are two important phases of fasting: the 8-hour period after your last meal (post-meal), and the next 8 hours, which is 16 hours after your meal (post-absorption). In principle, the first 8 hours mean the rest of your day after you have eaten. And the other 8 concern the morning period when you are fasting.

Prepare yourself mentally first. Do not go headlong while playing immediately. This is a drastic measure, keep that in mind. Ask yourself why you want to fast, and what your goal is.

To better support your fasting and allow your body to enjoy the benefits, you have two priorities: rest, and hydrate permanently!

Do not try to eat too much before starting the fast.

And you do not need to reduce your consumption before you start. The ideal is to do the young during a relatively calm period, in which you can protect yourself from any form of stress (during a leave for example).

If you play sports, prefer a partial teenager in which you will eat at least liquid foods , such as soups. And again, drink a lot of water.

Whatever your approach to fasting, you should talk to at least one health professional . Seeking advice from a naturopath is also a great idea, but it's important to talk to your doctor or doctor to monitor your progress.

Decide in advance the duration of the young

To know how to play effectively, you must decide on a fasting time. The effects of this approach vary according to the number of days and the regularity.

For example, you can play for 3 days , just enough time to react to the body and mobilize its resources. In this context, we can talk about fasting short . Your body will seek to fill primarily the lack of glucose in the brain (which is obtained with most proteins and amino acids in eggs, fish and meat).

You then have the option of prolonged fasting after the fifth day. This form of fasting can last several weeks. This is an extreme initiative that absolutely requires coaching with a professional. In this case too, it would be better to consider a partial fast with even a minimum of calories.

Make the young, a good approach provided you are careful!

Fasting can be offered from a therapeutic perspective , and it must be understood that it is not a cure. However, it is an approach that can be very effective if it is well organized and supervised, not only to help detoxify the body , but also to act as a preventive measure for certain treatments and diseases.

If you wish to try the experiment, we recommend you to surround yourself with professionals, and to opt for a fast of 3 days maximum.

Consider also a partial fast , with a minimum of caloric intake. And more than ever, your water consumption will have to be regular!

HOW LONG CAN A FAST CONTINUE

The usual autonomy of a healthy human being, without overweight, is of the order of thirty days. More in subjects who have a significant fat mass, beyond this period, which does not exceed six weeks without solid food, studies show that gluconeogenesis will regain importance, triggering a maximal metabolic alert that will constrain food recovery, failing which exhaustion and death may occur.

The human being is far from achieving in this area the performance of the penguin which can fast in the Antarctic for more than a hundred days

WHAT ARE THE RISKS OF FASTING THERAPY

According to the Ministry of Solidarity and Health, doing the fasting can be dangerous if you are not supervised with health professionals:

We have seen at best such inconveniences as migraines and discomfort. It is known that feeling hungry can cause you to faint, especially if you have slept little the night before.

A poorly supervised fast can also lead to heart problems, which represents a risk of mortality. This kind of risk can normally be caused after 1 to 2 weeks without solid food.

We can also see various deficiencies that will weaken the bones, as well as concerns of inflammation.

It must be understood that fasting is a drastic step, which upsets your body and pushes it to draw on its resources. Thus, fasting can be particularly extreme for children, growing teenagers, the elderly and, of course, pregnant women.

It has been estimated that fasting can also affect your fertility. In addition, if you are a woman, you will have to consider other side effects such as menstrual problems and worries if you are in menopause!

The strict fast (with only water) is not recommended for athletes, especially those of high level.

Contrary to what one might think, fasting does not particularly help to lose fat : this is especially the case for overweight people, because the excess food allows you to hold longer without caloric intake. .

On the other hand, the loss of water can be consequent with fasting! It is therefore of crucial importance to have a continuous water supply during your therapy.

There are many other consequences, so let's conclude with the most predictable effect: your mood. As a result of fasting, you may feel euphoric the first hours (or even the first 2/3 days). But past this moment, you will experience extreme mood changes , such as a tendency to be irritable, to make depression , or even paranoia.

Well, as you can see, not everything is rosy with fasting. To be sure to enjoy the benefits and avoid unpleasant surprises (and if you are determined to do so), there are several actions to follow:

CHAPTER TWO

SHOULD WOMEN FAST

There is some evidence about the possibility that intermittent fasting may not be as beneficial for women as it is for men. For example, one study showed that there is an improvement in insulin sensitivity in men, but that it worsened blood sugar control in women.

Although studies of human beings are not available on this subject, research in mice found that intermittent fasting can malnourish rats, masculinize them, make them infertile and cause them to lose their menstruation.

There are a large number of reports with anecdotes about women who lost menstruation when they performed intermittent fasting and recovered it when they returned to a normal eating pattern.

FOR THESE REASONS, WOMEN SHOULD BE CAREFUL WITH INTERMITTENT FASTING.

They should follow some different guidelines, such as facilitating the practice or stopping it immediately if they suffer from any problems such as amenorrhea (absence of menstruation).

If you have fertility problems and / or are trying to conceive, consider setting aside intermittent fasting for now. This eating plan is usually a bad idea if you are pregnant or breastfeeding.

SAFETY AND SIDE EFFECTS

Hunger is one of the main side effects in intermittent fasting. You may also feel weakness and the brain may not work as well as it usually does. It is possible that these effects are only temporary, since it takes time for the body to adapt to the new eating plan. If you have a disease, you should consult your doctor before attempting an intermittent fast.

This is very important if:

- Have diabetes
- Have problems with blood sugar regulation;
- Do you have low blood pressure;
- Take medication;
- It has less weight than normal;
- Has a history of eating disorders;
- She is a woman trying to get pregnant;
- Is a woman with a history of amenorrhea, or
- If you are pregnant or breastfeeding

That said, intermittent fasting has a great safety profile. There is no risk to stop eating for a few hours if you are healthy and have a general well-being.

INTERMITTENT FASTING FOR WOMEN

This is an appropriate technique for both men and women.

However, it is important to mention that women have a different metabolism and hormonal system that may conflict with their dietary regime.

Simply put, intermittent fasting that is too rigorous or performed improperly could cause hormonal alterations in the long run.

Despite that, and according to a recent study, when certain precautions are taken into account, fasting can be prescribed in women safely, and they can enjoy the same health benefits without significant adverse effects.

HERE ARE SOME RECOMMENDATIONS THAT WE CAN FOLLOW TO CARRY IT OUT SAFELY:

It is not recommended in pregnant, lactating women, or in those who have trouble sleeping and chronic stress.

All these conditions can lead to a hormonal imbalance initiated by an uncontrolled increase in cortisol. Similarly, there is not enough clinical data to recommend the method in pregnant women.

If you have or have had eating disorders, it is not a good option for you.

In women it is recommended alternately. It is not recommended that you do fasting for 16 hours every day without breaks.

The frequency of fasting per week should not exceed 3, and fasting protocols should not exceed 16 hours.

We can increase the number of fasting days to 4 for one week per month.

It is not convenient to start with 16-hour fasts immediately. Start with 10 hours, then increase the number of hours two by two until you reach 16.

On fasting days, it is advisable to perform light physical exercise to avoid increasing metabolic stress and cause a hormonal imbalance. Then, in the time you do not fast, take advantage of intense physical exercise.

On fasting days, drink plenty of fluids and always listen to your own body. Do not force yourself if you feel bad.

Use BCAA's supplements, which are especially useful before starting any fast exercise routine.

Arrow Recommended supplements

During morning abstinence, it is also possible to take nutritional supplements, and in many cases it could benefit and accelerate the achievement of your goals.

We could list multivitamins, antioxidants, omega 3, and protein supplements, especially BCAA's,

The Multivitamins increase nutrient availability, especially in certain geographic areas where there may be deficiencies.

Supplements Antioxidants are added to the benefits of intermittent fasting to decreasing the incidence of chronic diseases and hold off oxidative stress.

The omega - 3 is very useful in the ketogenic diet is a potent anti - inflammatory and improves cardiovascular health.

And BCAA's can be very useful for maintaining physical performance for those who carry out a daily exercise routine.

WHAT EFFECTS DOES FASTING HAVE ON WOMEN

If you are a woman, it is very likely that you went wrong dieting at least once - if not dozens of times - in your life. In fact, women experience intermittent fasting differently from men , so it is more complex for them to obtain results. Of course, it is still possible to achieve both psychological and physical benefits, but sometimes it requires a different approach.

For women, in particular, there are certain biological truths about fasting, so if we ignore them we will not be able to achieve our weight and health goals that we have set.

Fasting can be complicated, especially for women. In fact, intermittent fasting can cause a hormonal imbalance in women, to the extent that they are especially sensitive to any sign of hunger. If the body feels any sign of starvation it will start producing hunger hormones.

Therefore, when you stop fasting you may experience insatiable hunger. This is the way in which our body protects a potential fetus (even when we are not pregnant).

Many of us, determined women, ignore these signs of hunger. Or worse, we try to ignore them, but we fail and then we cannot avoid bingeing, then following another phase in which we eat below what is necessary, so that our body feels that risk of starvation again. And guess what: this can stop ovulation . Thus, in studies on animals it was noted that after two weeks of intermittent fasting, female rats stopped having menstrual cycles and their ovaries shrank; male rats saw their testosterone production decreased. It was also noted that female rats suffered insomnia in that process.

There are currently very few studies on animals that have analyzed the effects of fasting on women specifically, but studies on animals confirm our suspicion: intermittent fasting can significantly alter the hormonal balance of women, causing fertility problems.

WHAT CAN A WOMAN DO TO FOLLOW INTERMITTENT FASTING

If you notice that you are experiencing any of the symptoms previously collected while you are following an intermittent fasting program, you should stop completely. If the symptoms disappear and everything returns to normal within a couple of weeks, it is recommended to retry a moderate intermittent fasting program.

The question is how do we fast gradually without our hormones getting lost? For this it is considered not to fast every day , but on non-consecutive days so that our hormones are not disturbed. Thus, there is talk of intermittent fasting "crescendo", as you gradually become accustomed to your body to fast from time to time, until you reach the point that is right for you.

Therefore, it begins with a 12-16 hour fast for three days a week, but not consecutively, but separated from each other. During those three days you should focus on eating healthy for the period of time allowed. You can usually get this by simply skipping breakfast . During the days you are fasting, make sure you do shorter training sessions.

Another thing that I think really helps, but is not absolutely necessary, are the branched amino acids (BCAAs). These can maintain protein blocks in your system and therefore prevent muscle deterioration. In addition, they can help you mitigate the hunger that many of us experience in this process, especially during the first few days.

WHEN TO STOP INTERMITTENT FASTING?

If you notice any symptoms of hormonal imbalance such as those mentioned above, if you experience problems with your menstrual cycles or if fasting you think it could trigger an eating disorder, stop immediately, because intermittent fasting is probably not for you.

That said, I think that most of us, even those of childbearing age, could do this type of fasting without adverse effects but in a moderate way, provided that when you go to eat you do it in a healthy way.

INTERMITTENT FASTING FOR WOMEN OVER 50

Intermittent fasting is a fairly widespread type of diet among the population, in which the practice of long periods of fasting is encouraged to thereby promote weight loss. There are different studies that support this type of diet, however they are usually carried out in men and athletes.

Many women may be tempted to follow this nutritional strategy to lose weight, however, what effects can intermittent fasting have on them? Can you find it effective? Know why you should do intermittent fasting, what effects it can have on women and what you can do to try to avoid such effects.

TYPES OF FASTING

There is evidence that intermittent fasting may not be as beneficial for some women as it is for men.

A study in 2005 showed that after three weeks of intermittent fasting, blood sugar control in women worsened than men. Therefore here are the types of fasting that are most beneficial for women despite the fact that there are many other variations.

INTERMITTENT FASTING 12/12

Intermittent fasting 12/12 implies fasting for 12 hours and then having the freedom to eat for the remaining 12 hours of the day.

Fasting 12/12 used to be something natural and frequent in the past, before we began to implement the harmful habit of eating constantly. It was customary to have dinner at 7 in the afternoon and have breakfast the next day at 7 in the morning. But of course, this was when we lived a less modern and more structured life ... before we were tempted to fast food, frozen food, and microwaves.

This type of fasting is probably the best option for most women who want to start fasting since it is the simplest option and the one that requires less effort. This type of fasting will allow you to introduce fasting in a less intense and more gradual way to avoid causing a "shock" to the body and avoid side effects.

This option is the one that offers less health benefits, since your body needs a minimum of 12 hours to really enter a state where your hormones work together to start burning fat. Only at 12 hours of fasting is when glycogen stores begin to run out, insulin and glucose are at their lowest levels, and where glucagon hormone levels increase to help start the burning process of grease.

Although intermittent fasting 12/12 is the least beneficial, it may be a good option for women who have just begun to explore fasting and who wish to implement it daily.

If you are a beginner in this fasting or are looking for a fast that is not so restrictive and that is relatively easy to implement, this type of fasting may be a good option for you.

INTERMITTENT FASTING 16/8

Intermittent fasting 16/8 implies fasting for 16 hours and then having the freedom to eat for the remaining 8 hours of the day.

This type of fasting is probably the most popular option since it is neither too extreme nor too short a fast. As it is an average fast, you will receive more benefits than an intermittent 12/12 fast without going to extremes.

The 8-hour window for eating is also quite reasonable and therefore still allows you to have a relatively normal diet (3 meals a day with more than 4 hours difference between meals). This type of fasting can still be a good option if you want to do it daily but remember to start gradually.

INTERMITTENT FASTING 18/6

Intermittent fasting 18/6 implies fasting for 18 hours and then having the freedom to eat for the remaining 6 hours of the day.

It is here that we begin to enter the gray area for women because many women do not tolerate long fasts very well. Maybe your body type does tolerate it, but maybe that of many other women doesn't.

Sometimes short fasts are better for us women who want to burn fat. But if you decide to use this type of fasting, pay attention to see how your body feels!

Maybe it's not a bad idea to do this type of fasting from time to time ... maybe 2 times a week but in my personal opinion, I would NOT do it daily. The longer the fasts, the less frequent they should be.

INTERMITTENT FASTING 20/4

Intermittent fasting 20/4 implies fasting for 20 hours and then having the freedom to eat for the remaining 4 hours of the day.

This type of fasting is one in which you must eat larger meals but less frequently. Maybe you can make 2 meals a day with a difference of 4 hours between meals.

When we do longer fasts such as this intermittent 20/4 fast or a 24-hour fast, we run the risk of not eating enough food during the day since our window of time to eat is reduced to only a few hours and some people are Difficult to eat so much food in one sitting. That is why I do not recommend doing these types of fasting so frequently ... because they can become a type of low-calorie diet which will slow down our metabolism.

Remember when you practice intermittent fasting you should not reduce the amount of calories you consume in a day! The only thing you are trying to do is eat the same amount of food but in a shorter window of time.

Although I do not suggest intermittent fasting 20/4 daily (for women), it may be a good option to do it once every 2 weeks or once a month, as it offers many benefits that other shorter fasts do not offer.

For example, to induce the process of autophagy (the mechanism where the body removes damaged cells to regenerate newer and healthier cells), it usually takes 18-20 hours of fasting. Therefore, a 20/4 intermittent fast or a 24-hour fast can be excellent for keeping your cells young and healthy, and prolonging your life.

24 HOURS FAST

The 24-hour fast involves fasting for 24 hours and then making 1 meal after finishing the fast. This is a type of fasting that should only be done once or twice a month for a long time since it usually ends up being a day low in food and calories because many women find it difficult to eat so many foods in one meal. Besides, you can also take the risk of wanting to eat junk food or eat too much for having spent so many hours without eating and feeling very hungry.

This type of fasting can also interfere with our hormones and therefore can be more harmful than beneficial if done too often.

However, like intermittent fasting 20/4, the 24-hour fast also offers the benefits of autophagy. Therefore, I like to use this fast once a month to enjoy its benefits and avoid negative effects on my metabolism.

Again I remind you that the longer the fasts, the less frequently they should be done ... at least for us women.

Now that you know about the most popular and less harmful intermittent fasting for us women, let's move on to the 5 mistakes you should avoid when practicing fasting.

CHAPTER THREE

ERRORS WHEN STARTING INTERMITTENT FASTING

For example, start with very long fasts, but also do not drink anything during it (drinking water, all kinds of infusions, teas or coffees does not interrupt the process if you do not add sugars).

The big mistake is to end up obsessed with the hours and 'portions' of fasting , but the fault that worries professionals the most is an even simpler one: that this practice involves a binge-free bar. Few intakes, in a small number of hours, but of pizzas, hamburgers or ultra-processed

Even of alcohol. It is of no use, because how do you remember, if this combined practice is interpreted for a stage of fat reduction, what is not negotiable is the consumption of somewhat less fuel than is used. Therefore, the more information is consumed, you have about yourself and contrast with professionals, the better to obtain results

The main mistakes to avoid for successful intermittent fasting

Fasting to lose weight is not as simple as it seems. Indeed, some very common mistakes can ruin all your efforts and make intermittent fasting counterproductive.

Here is a list of the main mistakes to avoid for a successful fast.

Do not drink enough water

The elimination of metabolic waste and toxins requires sufficient hydration. In periods of intermittent fasting, this hydration must be even more important for the body to support periods of fasting and continues to function optimally. When fasting, thirst is often much less important. It is therefore imperative to pay attention to this point and drink at least 2 liters of water a day, distributing the intake over the day.

Eat twice more during periods of food intake

When fasting, it can be difficult to maintain a balanced diet during periods of food intake. Indeed, it is very tempting to jump on food, eat in larger quantities and turn to pleasure foods. This is a big mistake.

To take advantage of the health benefits of fasting, the quality of food during periods of food intake counts as much as the periods of fasting themselves, for example, meals rich in vegetables, whole grain cereals, lean protein and essential fatty acids should be promoted.

Set goals that are too difficult to reach

Fasting is a complicated exercise. To avoid missteps, it is recommended to go gradually and stay tuned to your body first. If you are fasting for the first time, try setting yourself goals in stages. Start by setting the time of your meal in the evening, back off your morning breakfast, etc. In this way, you can slowly increase the fasting time without rushing your body.

Fasting to lose weight only

Intermittent fasting is a way of life rather than a diet. Its purpose is not weight loss, although it contributes to it. Summing up the fast for this purpose alone can make it much more complicated. In fact, you run the risk of missing out on all the other benefits of fasting (physiological and psychological) and giving up more quickly. Also, it can be frustrating and confusing in the event of a food gap or weight loss that is considered too slow.

INTERMITTENT FASTING ERRORS

Before choosing what type of intermittent fasting to practice, it is VERY IMPORTANT that you know the ERRORS that can ruin your health and stagnate in weight loss.

Women are VERY different from men in matters of hormones and muscle mass, and therefore we must practice intermittent fasting in a different way. If you do not pay attention to these mistakes, you will fall into the same trap that many women fall into. You will end up frustrated and wondering why it doesn't work for you or why you feel worse than when you started. So let's move on to the mistakes that women make when implementing intermittent fasting.

Error # 1

DO NOT START GRADUALLY!!! If you are not accustomed to making long and sudden fasts you get into a fast for 16 - 24 hours, your body will experience a shock and your hormones will leave equlibrio. This can cause damage to your metabolism and instead of losing weight, you will end up frustrated and sick.

Begin to implement intermittent fasting gradually. Go gradually compressing the time window in which you eat and increasing the time window in which you fast.

For example, if you are used to having dinner at 8 pm and having breakfast at 6 am the next day, then this week try to have dinner at 6 pm and have breakfast at 6 am. This will increase your fasting window from 10 hours to a 12 hour window. Do it for 1 week and evaluate how you feel!

If you don't experience a lot of cravings, headaches or any other negative symptoms, then increase your fasting hours by 1 or 2 more hours the following week.

Error # 2

DO NOT LISTEN TO YOUR BODY! This is one of the WORST mistakes you can make. Many women choose to fast for 18 hours and although their body is shouting that they are hungry and even if they feel weak, if 18 hours have not passed, they do not eat.

What a fatal mistake! This is the only thing that will cause a slow metabolism and your body will cling to fat. That's why you should listen to your body at all times. Follow the method of intuitive intermittent fasting. Let your body guide you! Listen to the signals that your body gives you AT ALL TIMES!

If when you are doing an X hour of fasting you feel weak, you have headaches, you are hungry excessively, you feel that you are going to pass out or that you want to vomit ... ALL these are symptoms that you are exceeding yourself in the amount of hours of fast what are you doing and what do you need to eat?

This does not mean that you will never be able to fast for X hours. It just means that your body is not yet ready for such a long fast and that you have to start with a slightly shorter fast which you will gradually increase.

Error # 3

FASTING THE SAME AS MEN OR THE SAME AS OTHER WOMEN! As women it is VERY IMPORTANT to find the type of fasting that best fits our lifestyle and our body type. What works for men generally does not work for women. What works for me may not work for you!

We are all different and the fast that best suits your body may be different from that of your friend, neighbor, sister, etc. So try different schedules to see which one suits you best and which one fits with the activities you do daily. Try to be flexible.

For example, if you normally have dinner at 6 pm and have breakfast at 10 am the next day, but today you have an event with friends where you will have dinner until 8 pm, DON'T WORRY! You can have dinner at 8 pm and the next day just move your breakfast for noon or just fast a little shorter. NOTHING HAPPENS IF YOU MOVE THE SCHEDULE OR FAST A LITTLE LESS!

You do NOT need to fast for 16, 18, 20, or 24 hours EVERY day! You can vary the fasting hours you do daily. The hours of fasting that I do daily vary depending on how hungry I am or what activities I have that day. This gives me flexibility and allows my body to feel good at all times.

Error # 4

DO THE FAST TOGETHER WITH THE KETOGENIC DIET! DO NOT do intermittent fasting along with the ketogenic diet! It will be a tremendous shock to your body. If you have already practiced the ketogenic diet for some time, then you can start implementing intermittent fasting. However, if you are a beginner in the ketogenic diet, first let your body adjust to this new style of eating and then introduce intermittent fasting.

When you implement both at the same time, your body can resent so many changes and seek to protect itself by clinging to the fat and nutrients it is receiving instead of spending them freely.

Even I would recommend starting with the ketogenic diet first and then after a few months of having practiced the ketogenic diet, then add intermittent fasting. You will receive much more health benefits and weight loss with the ketogenic diet than with intermittent fasting.

This does not mean that intermittent fasting is not a fabulous tool for health and fat burning ... it just means that it is a more advanced tool that should be used to give an extra boost to our metabolism once It is in fat burning mode and on the way to better health.

THE HEALTH BENEFITS OF INTERMITTENT FASTING

Fasting would have many benefits on the body. Especially in our society where overeating and junk food are two common facts

Here are the main health benefits of fasting:

- Decreases insulin production and storage of fats and sugar in the body
- Stimulates destocking of fats
- Better control of food sensations
- Stimulates the secretion of growth hormone
- Improves physical and intellectual performance and decreases recovery time
- Promotes cellular regeneration
- Allows cleansing of the body and stimulates autophagy or self-cleaning function of the body by its own cells
- Decreases cellular oxidation and premature cell aging

- Prevents overweight and certain associated pathologies: cardiovascular diseases, diabetes, etc.

FASTING TO LOSE WEIGHT

Fasting to lose weight is the new trend. As mentioned above, the health benefits of fasting are numerous and very interesting. However, as part of a weight loss you have to be careful. Indeed, intermittent, unframed and poorly-led fasting can lead to more damage than profit. Fatigue, frustration, food compulsions, cravings, etc. are all negative effects that can put the body to the test.

To avoid them, it is necessary to seek medical advice before starting the fast and to be accompanied by food professionals. Also, keep in mind that fasting is not a diet but a way to eat. Weight loss should not be the only motivation at the risk of making things difficult and frequent mistakes.

INTERMITTENT FASTING TO LOSE WEIGHT

If you skip meals, you will create a caloric deficit and therefore lose weight, unless you offset your fasting with foods high in fat and sugar. Indeed, this method of feeding does not prohibit you to eat such or such food.

It's up to you to decide. According to some studies, intermittent fasting (if done correctly) not only reduces daily caloric intake, but also prevents the onset of type 2 diabetes. The body also learns how to better manage the foods eaten during pregnancy. food intake phase.

Studies have also shown that the combination of the 16/8 method and muscle development training (body weight exercises or additional weights) would reduce fat more effectively than bodybuilding alone. It also means that this method is especially fruitful combined with a regular exercise.

Caution: This type of diet is not recommended for people with diabetes, high blood pressure or pregnant or breastfeeding women. Before starting any type of diet, please consult your doctor first.

Fasting and exercise - how to combine the two

There are some important things to consider when combining fasting with exercise. If you are trying to lose weight, reduce your calorie intake moderately and aim for only 0.5 to 1% of body weight loss per week.

Incorporate muscle building sessions and lots of protein into your diet, about 25% or more of your total energy intake to help preserve your muscle mass. And try doing your workouts just before your biggest meal of the day. If you plan to combine intense training with the fasting phase, we advise you to consult a health professional first.

THE SOCIAL ASPECT OF INTERMITTENT FASTING

Fasting can be very effective in terms of weight loss. But have you ever thought for a second about the consequences on your social life?

Imagine: you're invited next Sunday to a birthday brunch. The breakfast buffet is covered with delicious muesli, fresh fruit, yoghurt, scrambled eggs, salmon ... All your friends enjoy this tasty breakfast. And you ? You sit next to them, a poor glass of water in their hands ... It's only 10 am, two hours before you can have your first meal of the day, because tonight you're invited to dine with friends. Rather frustrating, no? Try to plan fasting phases intelligently so that you can continue to have fun with your friends and family.

But as a rule, this type of diet does not leave much room for spontaneity! If this is something you care about, consider switching to another type of diet, such as the IIFYM diet, a diet where you can eat whatever you want as long as it fits into your nutrition plan. (distribution of different macronutrients)

WHAT TO DO IN CASE OF HUNGER?

Many people who try intermittent fasting complain of a permanent sensation of hunger, fatigue, exhaustion but also terrible cravings. This may seem logical, as you skip meals. But others also explain that this feeling of hunger disappears at the end of the first critical phase (which lasts about two days). And if the feeling of hunger becomes really unbearable, it is recommended to soothe with a cup of green tea or black coffee.

Intermittent fasting is certainly not for everyone. But this remains a very good way to lose fat. The important thing is to continue to eat balanced during the food intake and not to burgers, pizzas and fries to compensate.

KETOSIS AND INTERMITTENT FASTING: THE ULTIMATE AND WINNING MIX OF DIETS

Intermittent fasting and the ketogenic diet and they give us their opinion about its benefits and the problems that could result.

Ketosis is a normal metabolic state that is characterized by the elevation of ketone bodies in blood." By practicing intermittent fasting (16-24h) and / or reducing carbohydrates to the extreme, our brain begins to feed on fuel not ingested immediately . That is, it "uses ketone bodies" as the main source. Pull the reserves we want to burn.

Vázquez interprets this combination as "one more tool". Of course, he admits that his popularity is due to "many people lose fat easily" because this practice can give a greater benefit in the long term: control hunger.

Roberto Sánchez del Valle , the dietitian and nutritionist graduated from the Pablo Olavide

University best known for his Nufisa channel , agrees on that, but he warns of the opposite case: "this type of practice can lead to some Eating Disorder".

It refers to people psychologically "predisposed" and with outbreaks, such as the so-called 'binge eating disorder', which serve as an example to understand their limits.

On the chronological axis of evolution, until yesterday, we fasted. Therefore, according to Vázquez, as hunter-gatherers "we are not only adapted to periodic fasting, but incorporating them brings different benefits." In his program 'From zero to keto' , he describes the power of food control when doing a couple of cycles a year to 'ketone' our body.

TYPICAL DAY OF FASTING SPECIAL MENU

To help you build a day menu in practice, here is an example of a fasting special food plan. Fasting is the most popular and widespread method of intermittent fasting. This method consists of alternating a food intake period of 8 hours with a fasting period of 16 hours. Here, the last meal of the day is consumed before 20h and the first meal of the day is the next day lunch.

Lunch (at 12h)

Vegetable salad with walnut oil

150 to 200 g of meat, or substitute

200 g of green vegetables

200 g cooked whole starch

30 g of cheese

Seasonal fruit

Snack (at 16h)

Tea or infusion

Honey yoghurt

Oleaginous handle

40 g red fruit muesli

Dinner (before 8 pm)

250 g of vegetable soup

150 g of white fish or salmon, cottage cheese sauce and olive oil

200 g of cooked starch

Homemade fruit compote

2 squares of dark chocolate

To better match your habits, it is possible to set back the lunch hour and consequently the lunch time. The important thing is simply to keep a fasting period of 16h alternating with a food intake of 8h.

THE DIFFERENT TYPES OF INTERMITTENT FASTING

There is different way to apply intermittent fasting, I speak here of the best known.

THE LEAN GAINS METHOD (16H / 8H)

The method, from Martin Berkhan, was originally developed to optimize muscle gain by weight training and intermittent fasting. This is probably the most popular method today, it is the method I use and recommend you to test.

It consists in fasting during 16h and being able to eat during 8h. For this, just do not have breakfast. For example you finish dinner at 20h, you fast until the next day 12h minimum. Nothing prevents you from fasting more, if you wish.

THE WARIOR DIET

This method, invented by Ori Hofmekler is older, but very close to the Lean earnings method. However, here is no need to define a window of fasting and nutrition. We must follow his instinct.

The idea is not to eat enough in the morning and noon, then to take a big meal in the evening. Ori recommends physical activity during the "fasting" period. This method is not technically a fast as it allows to consume some food in small quantities during the day, for example a banana.

THE OMAD (ONE MEAL A DAY) ONE MEAL A DAY

This method is the strictest method of intermittent fasting, the hardest to follow in my opinion. It consists of taking only one meal a day, a big meal. The goal of this method is to prolong the fasting period as much as possible in a day. If you put an hour to eat the big meal, your fasting period lasts 23 hours.

THE METHOD 5: 2

This method was developed by Dr. Michael Mosley, it is largely thanks to his fasting documentary "eat, fast and live longer" that I tested intermittent fasting. The method is spread over the week. It breaks down into 5 days of normal feeding and 2 days of fasting. On fasting days you are only entitled to a mini meal of 500 kcal (a large salad).

THE 24hr FAST

This method is a francophone initiative. It's the combination of Thursday and fasting. It consists of one day of fasting per week, preferably on Thursday. You fast 24h or more.

For example you do not eat after dinner from Wednesday until breakfast on Friday morning. It represents a fast of 36h around. Or you fast until dinner on Thursday for a fast of 24h, to renew every week.

HOW TO PREPARE INTERMITTENT FASTING TO MAKE IT EASIER

We're not going to lie here, fasting is not easy, you're going to shit at first. But as with everything in life, good things are always on the other side of the effort.

I had the bad idea to throw myself as a barbarian in the fast, I explain: I went from a standard diet of three to four meals a day and a lot of sweet stuff in all that, at 20h of fasting by days and almost more added sugar. My body was literally panicked.

I'm going to give you here some tips that will allow you to prepare your body, gradually to fast, so that the transition is sweet. All of these tips are going in the same direction, getting your body used to using fat as a source of energy.

By doing this, your body will naturally start burning your fat when you intensify your fast. The transition will last two weeks, but you can adapt these periods to the pace that suits you.

For example instead of two periods of a week you can do two periods of 10 days. If you feel that you will really have trouble for example, prolonging this period of adaptation will greatly help you.

FIRST WEEK

You need to do only one thing for the first week. In fact you have to stop doing one thing: take your breakfast. Why ? two simple reasons:

Continue the fast of the night : indeed every night we fast during our sleep. For example if you stop eating at 9pm and the next day you have breakfast at 7am, you already fast 10h without special effort.

The goal of skipping breakfast is to extend this fasting period from 10am to 4pm fasting. So in our example if your last meal ends at 21h just add 16h to know when you will eat the next day, 21h + 16h = 13h the next day, lets clarify here that nothing prevents you from lunch at noon, 11am or much later at 14h if it suits you best.

You really have to appropriate this method and adapt it to your lifestyle, you will increase your chances of success in the long term.

The other benefit of skipping breakfast is that you will naturally consume less sugar in your day. The classic French breakfast is stuffed with sugar. Bread, cereal, jam and milk are very sweet and will mount your insulin in the morning.

So continuing the fast of the night has a big additional positive effect that will allow you to burn fat and heal your metabolism

During this first week your body will gradually get into the habit of using your fat as a source of energy and it will produce more and more ketone bodies so that your brain functions optimally even without eating.

SECOND WEEK

During this second week you will continue not to have breakfast but, you will also apply two points that will help you to stabilize your sugar level all day and keep it at a relatively low level.

We stop the added sugars

This point is important. If you are about to start intermittent fasting to lose weight it's because your weight, shape and health are not optimal. Added sugars are largely responsible for this situation. You must realize it and internalize it.

It is inevitably hard to say that we will have to stop sugar to be healthy. So many good things contain sugar: chocolate, cakes, ice cream ... it's almost impossible to avoid added sugars. Instead of thinking in terms of deprivation you have to tell yourself that right now you are going to become demanding and you are only going to eat things that are really worth it.

For example a birthday cake, an exceptional pastry that you do not cross often. The goal is to get the added sugar out of your everyday life so that it becomes exceptional in every sense of the word. Let's be honest, the majority of the sweet things we eat are not exceptional, so reserve this little treat for exceptions that are worth it.

Even the sweetener, sweetener and aspartame

During the whole preparation period and during periods of fasting, it is strongly discouraged to consume sweeteners. Even if they are of natural origin. Here's why:

Sweeteners stimulate your body in the same way as sugar, hormonally. Your mouth feels sweet, your pancreas will produce insulin so your body can regulate your blood sugar level.

But a high level of insulin literally blocks the use of fat as a source of energy and therefore stops your weight loss. Since you have not consumed sugar your blood sugar level will drop and this will cause hunger at best and hypoglycemia in the worst case.

We starch poor starchy nutrients at lunchtime

The other point that will help you start intermittent

fasting gently is to stop nutrient-poor starchy foods in the afternoon: bread, pasta, rice, sweet potato, quinoa, wheat, spelled, other seeds and everything else. flour base.

Not only do these starchy foods bring you almost no micronutrients, but they also have the unfortunate tendency to boost your blood sugar level and at the same time your insulin.

Recommended starchy foods are legumes such as chickpeas, beans, lentils. Sweet potato, squash. These starches provide more nutrients than others, contain less sugar and are absorbed more slowly because they are rich in fiber.

The goal here is to remove starchy foods that are likely to vary your insulin too strongly after your lunch. This will have the effect of reducing your cravings, cava help you stay in "destocking" mode of fat and optimize your use of fat as fuel.

AM I OBLIGED TO ADOPT ALL THESE CHANGES TO FAST

Obviously no! These are tips that will really help you make the transition easier. If you think that "I just want to fast and it's out of the question to change my eating habits" is that it's not the right time to introduce all these changes, it's not a problem.

You can simply fast without changing your habits.

Fasting is already a healthy habit that you intend to introduce into your life. It's better to make a change than to feel overwhelmed by all the things we're supposed to do, like eating healthy or playing sports.

Once you have adopted fasting and you feel comfortable with this practice, you can try to introduce a new habit that will improve your health.

HOW TO AVOID THE INCONVENIENCE OF FASTING

I will be sincere with you, fasting is difficult at times. Especially at the beginning, hunger tends to diminish over time, but some side effects can make their appearance.

People react differently to lack of food. We are all different and the difficulties that you will encounter while fasting are probably different from those that I knew.

To avoid the galleys that I knew during the fast I propose you here some simple solutions, I think that they will help you to prevent the inconveniences related to the fasting.

Cramps

I always had cramps on my feet, at night when I fasted at first, it quickly got me drunk. So I took the time to understand the origin of this problem and to test several things to prevent cramps.

Cramps are caused by an imbalance of electrolyte in the muscles. In general it means a lack of magnesium and potassium and sometimes sodium.

I speak very often of insulin in this guide, this hormone is really ultra important. It also influences our ability to retain electrolytes such as magnesium, potassium, calcium and sodium. When the insulin level is low, which is the case with fasting, the kidneys retain much less minerals. We end up eliminating many more minerals in our urine than when insulin is higher. If you start fasting, here's how to avoid cramps:

The solutions

Just take half a teaspoon of pink salt from the Himalayas every morning. To dilute in a glass bottom of water, you can also take extra minerals in the form of capsules during your meals. It is strongly recommended to supplement magnesium, because more than ¾ people are deficient, so if you adopt intermittent fasting you risk aggravating this deficiency. Strong magnesium deficiencies can cause serious problems such as heart rhythm disorders, so do not take a risk, take your supplements.

The constipation

It's a little embarrassing to tackle this subject but it's really essential. Constipation can manifest itself with fasting, it is not systematic, but when it does, it can complicate your task and erode your motivation. Constipation in normal times can be caused by many factors, but if it is triggered only by adopting fasting without any other lifestyle changes, it signals the same thing as cramps: a lack of minerals.

Another counter intuitive point that can cause constipation during fasting is overconsumption of water and other drinks. Indeed, to fight against hunger you will probably drink a lot of water, and as explained above your kidneys do not hold the minerals, so you will empty your minerals because you drink too much water. Your body will try to recover as many minerals in your digestive system and it can lead to constipation.

The solutions

As for cramps, half a teaspoon of pink salt from the Himalayas every morning, I also advise you to increase your consumption of vegetables, rich in fiber, however it should not be done abruptly, as this can aggravate constipation. Finally, I advise you to season your dishes well with olive oil or butter, it helps to lubricate the digestive system.

It is necessary to drink between 1 and 2 liters of water a day, preferably well spread over the day. It is also necessary to drink regularly, strongly mineralized waters

Headaches

The majority of people who start fasting encounter this problem. It is difficult to identify the cause of headaches but generally following the tips below they will disappear quickly.

Before you start fasting, your brain carbons sugar, after a few days of fasting, your body will produce ketone bodies. These will replace much of the sugar in your brain. The good news is that ketone bodies are a much cleaner source of energy than sugar. So be patient during this period of a few days or your body adapts to your new way of life.

The solutions:

If you do not drink a lot, do it! You must drink at least 1.5l of water and other herbal teas a day. However, to avoid cramps and constipation I advise you not to drink more than 2.5 liters.

The other point not to neglect is sleep. The cleaning of the brain happens in the evening, lying down only. So to properly eliminate the waste of your brain sleeps more than 6 hours, and makes sure to go to bed before midnight

hypoglycemia

Hypoglycemia is a sharp drop in blood sugar

levels. The normal sugar level is between 0.63 gr and 1.1 gr per liter of blood. What you need to know is that you can have the symptoms of hypoglycaemia (weakness, convulsions, unconsciousness) while having normal blood sugar levels. Why ?

This happens especially if you have significant variations over a short period. If for example your sugar level, after a meal, goes from 1.5 gr to 0.9 gr quickly, you can have the symptoms of hypoglycemia while your blood sugar is normal.

The sharp increases in blood sugar are caused by sugars and, to a lesser extent, proteins. The sharp drops in blood sugar are caused by a strong production of insulin. Both are necessarily linked. How to avoid high blood sugar variations?

The solutions

The solution is simple and can be broken down into two points:

Limit added sugars and low carbohydrates to nutrients such as bread, paws, rice and potatoes. These carbohydrates do not bring you much in terms of nutrients and they quickly turn into sugar in your blood. We must know that in our blood we must at most have the equivalent of a teaspoon of sugar.

A bowl of rice contains about 10 teaspoons of

sugar, necessarily, your blood sugar will increase and your insulin will also increase and you will experience a strong variation in blood sugar.

Increase good fats. In fact, fats have a zero glycemic index, so they have no negative impact on blood glucose. So season your vegetables with olive oil, butter. Including fat will generally lower the glycemic index of your meal. What you absolutely must not do is continue to eat large amounts of carbohydrate and increase the amount of fat.

Finally, I must remember that you must do your best to eliminate refined sugars from your diet. Refined sugars are really the most likely to cause a big change in your blood sugar.

The deficiencies

This is one of the things that scares the most of the loved ones when someone launches into a fast. To reassure my wife, I took multivitamins for more than a month to make sure I did not miss anything.

This fear is legitimate because if during your fast you have a poor diet of micro nutrients, which is the case in our modern diet, you will probably be deficient. In the short term impacts are often invisible because our body will draw on its stocks, but in the long run it can pose serious health problems.

The solutions

The best solution is also the cheapest is to eat real foods rich in nutrients, especially vegetables. We are reminded every day that you have to eat five fruits and vegetables a day. This is really the minimum in my humble opinion.

Our generation eats less fruit and vegetables than our parents and we are surprised that our health is deteriorating visibly. Fruits and vegetables are really very beneficial to our health. They bring us the majority of the micronutrients we need.

To be sure to consume enough, I always take care to build my meals around vegetables. I fill my plate of vegetables, I add a portion of protein

CHAPTER FOUR

MYTHS AND REALITIES ABOUT WEIGHT LOSS

Losing weight is not only an aesthetic necessity, but it has also become a method to prevent chronic diseases and a host of health problems.

A classic example is the focus on breakfast and meal times.

Traditionally, breakfast is considered the most important meal, which regulates all the metabolism of the rest of the day. In fact, in many countries the popular saying is known that recommends breakfast as king, lunch as prince and dinner as a beggar.

There are studies that prove that those who eat breakfast earlier lose more weight. The human body is very ironic and the opposite is also true. Intermittent fasting , which in many cases involves skipping breakfast, is also an effective method of losing weight.

On the other hand, there is a custom among nutritionists to suggest 6 meals a day instead of three to lose weight. Obviously, they should be smaller and well planned portions for the diet to work.

However, when we go to the scientific literature, what really matters is not the number of meals or the hours between them, but the number of calories consumed throughout the day.

Distributing food in 6 meals a day helps avoid a binge, but at the same time it accustoms the body to feed approximately every 3 hours, which can lead to a bad choice if the impending feeling of hunger takes you off guard.

Simply put, there is no magic routine that works for everyone.

Instead, there are different methods to reduce your weight, and they can all be effective if carried out in the right way.

More importantly, depending on our goals, priorities and lifestyle, some weight loss strategies may be better for us than others. In the case of intermittent fasting, for many, it can be very simple, and what is better, it can be applied in combination with other diets for greater results

THE BODY FAT PERCENTAGE

Both groups have a BMI above 20 (20.6 vs. 20.2), with the team absence period having a lower body fat percentage than the group with normal periods (18.6% vs. 19.8%).

19 seems to be the magic number in terms of amenorrhoea, because both a BMI of> 19 and a body fat percentage of> 19% form the framework for a healthy female cycle in my research.

Just as too high, too low a body fat percentage (especially in women) is not healthy. So if you are affected by amenorrhea or irregular periods and want to get back to a healthy cycle, then ideally your body fat percentage should be anything between 20-25%. Exceptions prove the rule

THE CALORIE DEFICIT DURING THE DAY

The researchers examined both the overall energy balance of the athletes, as well as the energy balance per hour during the day. Interestingly, the overall energy balance was the same for both groups , so all athletes took in the same amount of energy as burned. However, Team Amenorrhoea had a significantly greater and longer calorie deficit during the day than the group with normal periods. The girls without a period thus spent a higher number of hours in a catabolic state.

The researchers concluded that the more hours we spend a day on women in a negative energy balance, the higher our cortisol level (the stress hormone) becomes, and the lower our resting metabolic rate (RMR), T3, and estrogen levels become.

INTERMITTENT FASTING AND HORMONES

Our hormone system is closely linked to our metabolism. Intervening in the metabolism, our hormone balance can be disturbed, which can have consequences for our fertility.

Such an intervention may be the withdrawal of food, because our diet is an important set screw in this hormone-metabolism system. If we get too little energy and nutrients that we need, as can be the case with fasting, that means stress for the body.

Already short-term fasting of only 3 days should be able to change the hormonal impulses with some women. The result: a low estrogen level, which can be expressed in insomnia, mood disorders, metabolic disorders, weakened bones and even in non-existent or irregular periods.

IS INTERMITTENT FASTING MESSING UP OUR HORMONAL SYSTEM

Does that mean that intermittent fasting upsets our hormonal system and is responsible for amenorrhea and infertility?

However, the fact is that we women have a very sophisticated hormone-metabolism system that can easily be disturbed. And that diets that do not provide enough energy and protein can negatively impact our fertility. This can include intermittent fasting, if you do not plan properly.

To be healthy, young and fertile, we need two things: estrogen and amino acids [4] (which we get from a high-protein diet) - in a steady supply , not as binge-eating as the Warrior diet. We can gladly leave that to the men's world.

HOW DOES INTERMITTENT FASTING AFFECT CELLS AND HORMONES

When fasting, many changes occur in the body at the cellular and molecular level. For example, the body adjusts to hormone levels to better store body fat. Cells also initiate important repair processes and changes in gene expression.

Here are some changes that may occur in the body during fasting:

Growth hormone (HC): Growth hormone levels soar and increase up to 5 times. This has benefits for weight loss and muscle gain, to name a few.

Insulin: Insulin sensitivity improves and levels decrease dramatically. The decrease in them makes it possible for body fat to be better stored.

Cellular repair: During fasting, cells initiate a cell repair procedure. This includes autophagy, when cells assimilate and eliminate old and dysfunctional proteins that are built inside.

Gene expression: There are changes in the function of genes related to longevity and disease protection.

These changes in hormonal levels, cell function and gene expression are responsible for the health benefits of intermittent fasting.

A VERY POWERFUL TOOL TO LOSE WEIGHT

Weight loss is the most frequent reason for people to try intermittent fasting.

By needing fewer meals, intermittent fasting tends to produce an automatic reduction in calorie intake. Additionally, intermittent fasting modifies hormonal levels to facilitate weight loss.

In addition to reducing insulin levels and increasing the growth of hormonal levels, it also increases the release of norepinephrine (norepinephrine), a hormone that promotes fat reduction.

Due to these changes in hormones, short-term fasting could increase the metabolic rate between 3.6 and 14 percent. By assuming help to eat less and burn more calories, intermittent fasting causes weight loss by modifying both sides in the Harris-Benedict equation.

Studies have shown that intermittent fasting can be a very powerful tool for weight loss. A 2014 study found that this eating plan can cause between 3 and 8% of weight loss in about 3 to 24 weeks, which is a very significant amount compared to most studies for weight loss. .

According to the same study, people also lose between 4 and 7% of the waist, which indicates a significant loss of harmful fat in the abdomen, which appears around the organs and causes diseases.

Another study showed that intermittent fasting causes less muscle loss than more standardized methods of caloric restriction.

However, keep in mind that the main reason for

this success is that intermittent fasting helps you eat fewer calories overall. If you binge or eat compulsively during periods when you can eat calories, you will not lose any weight.

WHAT ARE THE SIGNS OF A HORMONAL IMBALANCE IN WOMEN

- Fatigue
- Depressed mood
- Swelling.
- Headache.
- Irregular menstrual periods.

WHAT CAN WE DO DURING THE FASTING PERIOD TO COPE WITH HUNGER

Ideally, the period of fasting coincides, in part, with the hours we spend sleeping, so that we spend part of that time sleeping and without feeling that hunger call that in the first days you may feel at not being used

But if for the reasons that are those hours that we spend sleeping are few, another tip is that part of that fast coincides, for example, with your workday to keep you busy and that time passes faster and you do not enter so many want to eat. Obviously, if you have a stressful job, the fasting protocol may not be a good idea, since stress makes good friendships with hunger and food , and we could end up committing some "atrocity" against our body.

CHAPTER FIVE

WHAT IS INTERMITTENT FASTING

It is a dietary regimen based on extending the period of night fasting for 16 hours or more. We talk about fasting to refer to a period of time greater than 8 hours in which we do not eat any food or drink with energy load.

This technique is called intermittent fasting because it alternates fasting periods with feeding phases in which we program the necessary nutrients to keep our energy and health levels in optimal conditions.

Intermittent fasting is the process of cycling between eating and not eating. Fasting intermittently loses weight, but is not a diet plan, but a lifestyle choice to enjoy some incredible health benefits.

Intermittent fasting (AI) is currently one of the most popular health and fitness trends in the world.

People usually put it into practice to lose weight, improve their health and simplify their lifestyles. Many studies have shown that it can have very positive effects on the body and brain, and that it can even extend life.

Intermittent fasting (AI) is a dietary pattern that is characterized by alternating periods of fasting and feeding. It does not detail the foods we should eat, but it does specify when we should eat.

In this regard, it is not considered a conventional diet, rather it could be described as an eating plan. The most common intermittent fasting methods involve fasting for 16 or 24 hours, twice a week.

Fasting has been carried out throughout the evolution of the human being. The ancestral hunters and gatherers had no supermarkets, refrigerators or food available throughout the year and sometimes they couldn't find anything to eat.

As a result, humans developed the ability to endure without eating for large periods of time. In fact, fasting from time to time is more natural than eating 3, 4 (or sometimes more) meals a day every day.

Fasting is also usually done for spiritual or religious

reasons, such as in Islam, Christianity, Judaism and Buddhism.

Intermittent fasting IS NOT A DIET! It is a tool that you can use to repair metabolic problems, hormonal imbalances, and insulin resistance, which are the factors that usually prevent women from losing weight.

So the main function of this tool is to primarily improve health, with the side effect of loss of body and abdominal fat.

Intermittent fasting says nothing about what foods to eat but rather when you should eat them. Intermittent fasting does not imply eating less. That is, you should consume the same amount of food (maintain your calorie intake) that you normally consume in one day but during a restricted time window. So you will have to eat larger meals for a shorter time. EYE! This is one of the biggest mistakes women make when practicing intermittent fasting.

Intermittent fasting involves alternate cycles of fasting and feeding. That is, divide the day into 2 time windows, a time window where you are going too fast and the other time window where you are going to eat.

In fact, most people already fast while we sleep. These 6-10 hours where we sleep are our fast window. By having our breakfast, we break our fast and enter the window of time to eat.

However, if you want to use fasting to improve health and delay aging, it should be practiced in a window of a minimum of 12 hours. That is, to begin receiving the benefits offered by intermittent fasting, it is essential that you fast for at least 12 hours.

It is here that different types of intermittent fasting come in.

Although intermittent fasting can help you lose weight, the reality is that this tool should be used mostly to improve health and as a side effect to enjoy weight loss.

Like all women we are different, we have different genes, different habits, and different lifestyles, some could lose more weight than others. There is NOT a magic number that applies to all women. The amount of weight you could lose will depend on your body, your metabolism and your health. What's more, you might not lose weight.

If you are a woman who has many health problems, maybe you could not lose an ounce of fat because the priority for your body at this time is not to lose weight but to restore your health. Therefore, use this tool as it really is, a health tool to be younger, healthier and have a longer life.

Intermittent fasting is an advanced tool that

should be used to give an extra boost to our metabolism once it is already in fat burning mode and on the way to Better health

BENEFITS OF INTERMITTENT FASTING

While not all diets work for everyone, it has many benefits that may interest you.

Many people have managed to incorporate these schedules into their daily routine and have not gone back for years.

Some of the commonly reported benefits are:

ACCELERATE YOUR WEIGHT LOSS

It is the reason why you would bother to change your eating rhythm, and it is worth it. This enhances weight loss by promoting the oxidation of fats for energy.

At the same time, it is very possible that you end up consuming fewer calories in two daily meals than in six, although they are very loaded.

IMPROVES INSULIN SENSITIVITY

Insulin resistance is a very common problem in people who are overweight and obese, and it is the prelude to diabetes.

This happens because, as there is no such constant stimulus and insulin peaks so frequent, your body counteracts what it perceives as a decrease in insulin secretion by increasing the receptors in the cells. Thus, the next time your pancreas secretes insulin, it will not need to release so much of this hormone for it to have the desired effect.

REDUCE TRIGLYCERIDE AND CHOLESTEROL LEVELS

Some studies have shown that it improves blood lipid levels without affecting the degree of good cholesterol (HDL). This in turn can reduce cardiovascular risk, decreasing the incidence of atherosclerosis, coronary heart disease, and other health problems.

REDUCE THE INCIDENCE OF SOME NEUROLOGICAL PROBLEMS

Recent studies have also found the relationship between intermittent fasting and decreased neurological risk, especially neurodegenerative diseases such as Alzheimer's, other types of senile dementia, and Parkinson's.

PROMOTES AUTOPHAGY - CELLULAR REPAIR

The relationship between fasting and neurodegenerative diseases, such as Alzheimer's, is recognized. Studies in animal models have shown that abstinence from food improves processes of cellular autophagy, through which the cell is able to degrade and recycle waste materials so that they do not accumulate in brain tissue, causing long-term problems.

In this sense, more than aesthetic benefits, it can have a profound neuro-protective effect.

REDUCE THE MARKERS OF INFLAMMATION

A recent study that evaluated the effect of feeding time on systemic inflammation and showed that increasing the hours of overnight fasting results in an 8% reduction in C-reactive protein, a marker of systemic inflammation associated with chronic inflammation and at breast cancer

The effect was more pronounced in women who consumed less of the calories in their last meal of the night, with which we can conclude that far from causing metabolic imbalances, it can become an ally to avoid systemic inflammation associated with chronic diseases.

HEALTHIER AND SIMPLER LIFESTYLE

Healthy eating is very simple, but it can be very difficult to maintain. One of the main obstacles is all the work required to plan and cook healthy foods. Intermittent fasting can make things easier, since you don't need any plans, or cooking, or cleaning after each meal as before.

For this reason, intermittent fasting is very popular among life-hackers (people who, with small tricks, manage to be more productive and efficient in all aspects of their lives), since it improves their health while simplifying their style of life.

DECREASE HUNGER

Beyond in the field of hormones and metabolism, it has been associated with hormonal changes in the levels of leptin and ghrelin, the two key hormones for the control of hunger and satiety.

This modulation is achieved gradually, which explains the reason why intermittent fasting for 16 hours becomes easier to tolerate over time.

Far from making us feel more hungry, it is a tool to restore the balance between hunger and the feeling of satiety.

YOU SAVE TIME AND MONEY

The idea of 6 meals a day sounds interesting until you start applying it. There comes a time when you stop living your life to stay cooking throughout the day, or you have to spend a whole afternoon making food for several days if you want to have more time for yourself. Not counting the planning and spending that this requires.

Instead, you should only worry about two main meals throughout the day. It makes your life simpler and works well to reduce your weight.

There have been many studies on intermittent

fasting, both in animals and in humans. These studies have shown that they can have great benefits for weight and health control of our body and brain and could even extend life.

Detoxification, purification, cleaning can be called in many ways, but ultimately the balance between eating and not eating. To make the idea clearer, we will refrain from eating for a certain period of time and then talk about having a regular meal for different periods depending on the type of fasting chosen.

There are many benefits of fasting:

- Insulin resistance: Intermittent fasting can reduce insulin resistance and lower blood sugar by 3 to 6 percent. In addition, it can accelerate insulin levels by 20-31%, which should protect against type 2 diabetes.
- Inflammation: Some studies have shown reductions in inflammation indicators, a key factor in many chronic diseases.
- Heart health: Intermittent fasting may reduce LDL (bad) cholesterol, blood triglycerides, indicators of inflammation, blood sugar and insulin resistance; All of them risk factors for heart disease.
- Cancer: Animal studies suggest that intermittent fasting may prevent cancer.
- Brain health: Intermittent fasting increases brain hormone (brain-derived neurotrophic

factor or FNDC) and may help in the growth of new cells. It could also protect against Alzheimer's.
- Anti-aging: Intermittent fasting can extend the life of mice. Studies have shown that fasting mice lived between 36 and 38% more.
- Keep in mind that research is still in the early stages. Many of the studies were small, short or carried out on animals. There are still many questions to be answered in studies of higher quality in humans.
- This is not a cost, you can save by reducing your daily meals.
- It is not a meal that complicates your life, but rather the opposite.
- You can fast anywhere, but this is not always possible on some diets.
- You can eat the necessary (healthy) food.
- Improved cognitive function.
- Promotes fat loss
- Improves insulin sensitivity
- Accelerate the metabolism
- Kill the bad bacteria found in the colon
- Promote a longer life
- Decrease hunger
- Decrease cravings
- It improves brain function
- It improves the immune system
- Fights cancer cells that feed on glucose
- It can reverse diabetes
- Improve fatty liver

- Improves neurodegenerative disorders
- Help with cell regeneration and repair to keep you younger
- Normalize blood pressure
- Improve allergies
- It gives our digestive organs a rest
- Improve lipid parameters

the benefits of intermittent fasting are amazing. That's why intermittent fasting is gaining such popularity recently. And it's not just because it's a fashion trend but because it's really beneficial.

INTERMITTENT FASTING AND THE MYTH OF BREAKFAST

The word breakfast refers to the morning meal, which takes us out of the night fast. Hence the ending "des" fasting

Certainly, the first food that opens the day and ends the fast is very important, no matter what time it is consumed.

That is why, the first thing we must do to understand it is to eliminate the myth of breakfast: Waking up without breakfast and going straight to a snack or lunch does no harm to anyone or cause any health problems.

Our body is accustomed to fasting. It is programmed for such a thing. It was not until recently, with the era of industrialization, that we began to receive all kinds of easily prepared foods that make it easier to eat something right after getting out of bed.

Instead, our ancestors had to fight for their food from early in the morning, and many times it could begin to get dark before having their first main course of the day.

So, making the decision to skip some meals on purpose does not have to hurt anyone.

On the contrary, we have genes programmed for it. Intermittent fasting is just that. It is not a diet in which you select your nutrients during the day. Rather, it is a dietary pattern or feeding schedule in which you will assign the foods you plan to consume during the day.

There are different types of fasting, each with its schedules and recommendations. Although, the most common are two: the 16/8 protocol and the 24-hour protocol, in which you extend the fasting period by 16 and 24 hours respectively.

METHODS FOR INTERMITTENT FASTING

There are many different ways to perform intermittent fasts and they all involve the division of the day or week to perform periods of feeding and fasting.

During periods of fasting, you can eat little or nothing. These are the most popular methods:

The 16/8 method: It is also often called the Lean Gains protocol and involves skipping breakfast and eating food for 8 hours, for example, between 1 and 9 in the afternoon. Therefore, a 16-hour fast is performed.

Fast eat-stop-eat: It involves a 24-hour fast, once or twice a week. For example, skipping dinner and not having dinner until the next day.

5: 2 diet: With this method, you can only consume between 500 and 600 calories on two consecutive days a week, but you can eat normally for the other 5 days.

If you reduce your calorie intake, all of the above methods should cause weight loss, as long as you do not compensate for fasting with meals that are much larger than normal.

Many people believe that the 16/8 method is the most simple, sustainable and easy to endure, so it is the most popular.

INITIATION TO INTERMITTENT FASTING

Most likely we all have done many intermittent fasts throughout his life and does not know. If you have had dinner, you have gone to bed, and have not eaten until lunch the next day, you have probably fasted for more than 16 hours.

Some people eat this instinctively, since they

simply are not hungry in the morning. Many people believe that the 16/8 method is the simplest and most sustainable, so you should try to practice this first.

If you believe that fasting is easy and feels good while doing so, try to make longer fasts, such as 24 hours 1 or 2 times a week (eat-stop-eat fasting) or eat between 500 and 600 calories for 1 or 2 days a week (5: 2 diet).

Another approach is to simplify fasting when convenient. You just have to skip meals every now and then not hungry or time to cook. You do not need to follow a structured intermittent fasting plan so you can get your benefits. Experiment with different approaches, find what suits you best and adjust it to your plan.

Should I try?

Intermittent fasting is not something that everyone needs to do. It is simply one of the main lifestyle strategies that can improve your health. If you eat real food, exercise and sleep the necessary hours, you don't have to worry about anything.

If you do not like the idea of fasting, you can ignore this article without any problem and continue with the lifestyle that is most suitable for you. At the end of the day, there is no single definitive solution for everyone when it comes to nutrition. The best diet you can do is the one you can sustain in the long term.

Intermittent fasting is very good for some people, but not for others. The only reason to discover the type of fast that suits you best is to try them all. If you feel good while fasting and think it is a sustainable way of eating, you may have found a fantastic tool to lose weight and improve your health.

CHAPTER SIX

HOW TO DO INTERMITTENT FASTING: FIRST STEPS TO START

After counting your macronutrients and knowing what you are going to eat during the day (after choosing between the Ketogenic diet and the anti-inflammatory diet that we propose), what remains is to calculate the schedule of your different meals taking into account fasting periods.

For this, two types of protocol have been devised, one of 16 and another of 24 hours. Ideally, start with the 16-hour protocol, taking into account that it is not so complicated and many of us have probably already done something like this in the past.

Subsequently, we will increase fasting hours and adapt them to our circumstances, work schedules and pace of life.

Protocol 16/8

This type requires lengthening the fast for 16 hours a day and feeding for the remaining 8 hours. Said in this way, it seems too much to have to endure 16 hours with hunger, but it is not necessarily so. Let's say you go to sleep at 10pm after having your last meal of the day at approximately 8 at night. You will complete your 12 hours of fasting at 8 in the morning, but if you only make the effort to skip a breakfast until 12 noon, you will have already completed your 16 hours without making too much effort.

It's something so easy that some people do it without even planning it. Seen that way, even you could have done some intermittent fasting without realizing it. Now, you can also take advantage of bedtime to skip a dinner. For example, if you make your last meal of the day at 4pm you will have 12 hours of fasting at 4 in the morning and already at 8am you can have breakfast having completed your 16 hours. Of course, it helps a lot if your last meal of the day is very substantial and is the one that leaves you most satisfied.

24 hour protocol

When you have more experience, it will be easier to extend your fasting period beyond 16 hours. You will notice as you progress through intermittent fasting that the sensation of hunger will gradually decrease and it will be easier to comply with a 24-hour protocol. There is not much to explain in this space. Simply, if your last meal of the previous day was at 9pm, your first meal of the next day should be at the same time of night. In this case, you should prepare your body before performing a 24-hour protocol.

Start by extending the fast for 18 hours and then 20 hours to test how your body reacts and how you feel. You must do this on separate days, maximum 2 times per week.

Although there is not much to explain about what you have to do during fasting periods, a frequent question has to do with fluid consumption. During this time you can consume water and drinks with little or no caloric index such as coffee or tea, as long as they have no sugar, dairy, or any other aggregate.

It should be noted that, especially while you get used to it, you may at some point feel very hungry, stress and mood swings. If this happens, eat something. Nothing will happen to you. The adaptation process could be gradual and it is best to keep trying and listen to your own body.

Although, you have to be aware of yourself and find the balance between listening to your body and being too condescending and permissive

CALENDARS FOR INTERMITTENT FASTING

Just as there are different fasting protocols, there are also different programs or calendars that we can follow.

We do not have to follow a 16-hour fast every day

of the week, much less can we do 24-hour fasts so followed by each other.

So there are 3 ways to schedule your fast: weekly, alternate, and daily.

WEEKLY FREQUENCY

It is the most appropriate strategy to start and test how our body responds. Some people start once a month or once every two weeks.

It all depends on our body, our habits and lifestyle. The benefits of fasting are maintained. It could be a good idea weekly for 16 hours and gradually increase the frequency.

Similarly, you can combine the weekly protocol with the 24-hour protocol if you have more experience with the method. The 24-hour weekly method is a good option for those who want to increase muscle mass by keeping their weight off or decreasing their body fat percentage. By doing so, we will not be in danger of entering catabolism and we can reduce our weight in a safe way.

ALTERNATING FREQUENCY

You can choose to increase the frequency by practicing it one day yes, one day no. By alternating days with fasting and days without it you will achieve a more gradual adaptation process and increase the fasting period during the week.

Again, they can be fasting for 16 or 24 hours. The only recommendation is to avoid a frequency greater than 3 times per week if you decide to fast for 24 hours. This approach is more focused on weight loss, although it is also appropriate for those who have an exercise routine and want to increase muscle volume in the process.

DAILY FREQUENCY

It is also called the Lean Gains model, the original model from which others derive.

Obviously, in this case only the 16-hour protocol only applies.

It could be the final stage of the previous two, and requires skipping a meal a day every day, without rest. There are modified models in which you can take two days off, usually during the weekend, as long as you keep your diet and keep eating healthy. Daily fasting is a model clearly designed to lose weight, but it is not inappropriate for those who want to gain muscle.

There are many experiences of those who have achieved good gains while reducing their body mass percentage. What you should keep in mind is to maintain a good protein intake to maintain muscle volume.

COMBINED FREQUENCY

If you want to go one step further, you can

combine the daily intermittent fasting of 16 hours with a weekly or alternate 24-hour fast.

As a general recommendation, this approach is much more restrictive and should only be used by those who already have several months of experience.

In this case, the 24-hour fast is recommended weekly, maximum twice a week. This approach is clearly for weight loss, and it should be emphasized that during the 24-hour fast days it is convenient not to perform too strenuous physical activity and always listen to our body.

WHAT YOU SHOULD TAKE INTO ACCOUNT BEFORE STARTING

While it is true that it is a good technique to lose weight, it is not the panacea or the solution of evils completely.

The adaptation process can be difficult for some, and in many cases it will be difficult to adapt this new diet to your lifestyle, your responsibilities, your work, training schedules, among others.

It will depend a lot on who lives with you, if you have support to do so, and if you have other responsibilities that may be affected.

Although, many people have managed to adapt their lives to intermittent fasting with a little patience and perseverance

You should keep in mind that the transition between eating 6 times a day and reducing the frequency to two main meals can be difficult.

Most of us who begin this method experience hunger, some feel a decrease in their energy levels, ability to concentrate, and even bad mood during the first few days.

The important thing about it is that it won't last forever. You will generally be able to adapt within a maximum of one or two weeks, unless there is a basic metabolic or nutritional problem.

Later, you will realize that your desire to eat will decrease instead of increase, and it is then and only then that you will start trying the 24-hour protocols.

INTERMITTENT FASTING WITH KETOGENIC DIET AND ANTI-INFLAMMATORY DIET

By incorporating it, you will not be making changes in what you eat but in the schedule in which you take food. However, for it to function properly, it must be associated with an appropriate regimen.

It would not make sense to eat excessively and unhealthily and then fast for 16 hours. One of the most commonly used diets in intermittent fasting is the ketogenic diet .

In fact, fasting accelerates the goals by facilitating and accelerating ketosis. Another suggested regimen for those who wish to take this process is the anti-inflammatory diet , which is a little more flexible than the ketogenic one, although it is more focused on reducing inflammation, maintaining weight loss as a secondary benefit.

The ketogenic diet requires consuming a very low amount of carbohydrates and increasing the consumption of healthy fats to get energy from them. The goal is for the food to contain 75% fat, 20% protein and only 5% carbohydrates.

For its part, the anti-inflammatory diet requires a decrease in the moderate carbohydrate count, reducing these to 40% and keeping fats and proteins at a rate of 30% each.

Whichever dietary option we choose, the most important thing is to maintain a dietary intake and a favorable calorie count, whatever the distribution of food throughout the day.

WHAT TO DRINK DURING THE FASTING PERIOD.

Although the idea is not to eat for a prolonged period, we can drink liquid, and what is more, it is advisable to do so. Liquid intake should not stop at any time of the day , and it can help reduce the feeling of hunger.

However, not all drinks are appropriate.

The drinks to choose during fasting periods must be without carbohydrates or calories, or with a very low level.

Water is the first and most obvious liquid allowed, but we can also consume coffee or tea, as long as it is not sweetened, much less served with milk or some other aggregate.

YOUR CONTRAINDICATIONS

It may not be the best option for all people equally.

It should be avoided if you have been diagnosed with any type of eating disorder, or in case of suspicion. In these cases, it could exacerbate the problem and do more harm than good.

Similarly, if you constantly suffer from hypoglycemia, it could regulate your insulin levels and improve the condition or have the opposite effect and cause severe blood glucose problems.

Therefore, in case of hypoglycemia and diabetes, it would be convenient to ask your doctor and maintain close control, especially at the initial stage and while your body adapts to your new diet.

CAN YOU EAT OR DRINK SOMETHING DURING INTERMITTENT FASTING

A popular misconception is that you can afford to

eat or drink certain drinks during the fast. To get all the health benefits of intermittent fasting, you should restrict the consumption of ALL TYPES of caloric foods during fasting. The point of fasting is to give our body a break from food! Therefore, you MUST NOT EAT ANYTHING!

But you can still consume non-caloric drinks because they will not increase your blood glucose levels and insulin release and therefore will not break your fast.

THE TYPE OF DRINKS THAT CAN ITSELF CONSUME DURING INTERMITTENT FASTING ARE AS FOLLOWS:

- Water
- Sparkling water
- Mineral water
- Coffee black pure without milk or cream (be careful if you decide to consume coffee because caffeine can cause damage to the metabolism of women)
- tea herbs / infusions

All these drinks should be pure and without sweeteners. There is debate about the use of stevia, erythritol or monk fruit during fasting and it is not known with certainty if they break the fast. But it must be taken into account that these ingredients must still be metabolized by the body despite not increasing blood glucose levels, therefore, there is reason to think that they can interfere with fasting.

That is why I prefer not to use them or drink anything (including coffee), except water or herbal teas / infusions during my fast.

WHAT TO EAT AND WHAT TO NOT EAT

It seems clear that running such high speeds to lose weight do not mean that you can eat excess calorie food during the period of food intake. You can eat whatever you like, but you can eat to some extent. Pizzas, prepared meals, or boat stews don't seem optimal.

Nor does it mean that you cannot take anything during a fast. Therefore, you can drink just coffee, sugar-free gum, water, infusions, or products that don't add extra calories every day.

In any case, it is always best to match fasting time and sleep time so that you do not think about food and do not properly respect the fasting protocol, but this is not always possible, especially for the first time.

WHAT TO EAT AFTER INTERMITTENT FASTING

One of the main reasons why intermittent fasting is practiced is to eliminate insulin resistance. Therefore, it is clear that to break the fast we need to eat foods that do not cause blood sugar spikes to avoid perpetuating insulin resistance.

Therefore, here you are realizing how important it is to break your fast with foods that are low in carbohydrates. Avoid foods high in carbohydrates such as flours, foods with sugar, starchy vegetables, cereals, grains, etc.

Your first meal should consist of a little protein, healthy fats and fiber from green vegetables (or low-carb vegetables) to break your fast. You can include fruit as long as it is a low carb fruit such as berries. If you decide to eat any other fruit higher in carbohydrates, then make sure it is in small quantities.

The key here is to experiment with your body to see what makes you feel good.

For example ... in the following video I show you one of my breakfasts to break the intermittent fast. I decided to include some fruit in this breakfast because I realized that my body likes a little fruit in the morning, especially when I combine it with green vegetables full of fiber, protein and healthy fats.

But if you feel tired and sleepy after eating fruit, then it means that your body does not tolerate fruits or foods a little higher in carbohydrates after fasting. So for the next try a breakfast based on eggs, vegetables and avocado.

The point here is that you should always listen to your body and make the necessary adjustments until you find what works for you!

EXAMPLES OF WHAT YOU COULD EAT TO BREAK YOUR FAST.

OPTION # 1:   Scrambled eggs with mushrooms and sweet peppers stewed in butter or with slices of avocado.

OPTION # 2:   Strawberry smoothie made with 1 cup of almond milk, 2 scoops of hydrolyzed collagen , 1/2 cup of strawberries, 1 tablespoon of hemp seeds , and a tablespoon of coconut oil .

OPTION # 3:   Pudding made with chia seeds , coconut milk, unsweetened grated coconut, raspberries, and some stevia or maple syrup.

INTERMITTENT FASTING AND EXERCISE

Is it wrong to exercise on an empty stomach?

Contrary to popular belief, exercising on an empty stomach can be very beneficial and quite safe. Exercising during an intermittent fast can help you burn a lot more fat. However, before exercising on an empty stomach, the following precautions must be taken into account.

If you are a beginner in intermittent fasting or

have a diet that is mostly focused on carbohydrates as fuel, then you should be more careful when exercising fasting, as your body is still used to burn glucose instead of fat.

It is here where you may experience dizziness, nausea or feel weak when exercising intensely on an empty stomach. The good news is that with less intense exercise during intermittent fasting you can prevent many of these symptoms and even burn fat.

As your body gets used to fasting, your body will feel more lucid and more energetic, which will make it easier for you to exercise while fasting, the most important thing when exercising fasting is that you listen to your body at all times!

If you feel dizzy, stop exercising immediately and eat something small before continuing to exercise. Take a break if you feel weak. Reduce the intensity of your exercise if you don't have enough energy.

As long as you are consuming enough nutrients during your feeding window and listening to your body when exercising, everything will be fine!

CHAPTER SEVEN

WHAT IS KETOSIS

The ketosis is a metabolic state of the organism caused by a deficiency in the intake of carbohydrates, which induces catabolism of fat in order to obtain energy , generating compounds called ketone bodies , which break down fats in shorter chains, generating Acetoacetate that is used as energy by the brain (in fasting states it provides 75% of the energy) and the rest of the organs of the human body.

In this way, the body stops using carbohydrates as a primary source of energy , replacing them with fats .

In the state of ketosis the body is able to oxidize fat easily, including the individual's own reserves. That is why there are many slimming diets that induce this state in order to reduce body fat.

FEATURE OF KETOSIS

During that process, as in so many other metabolic processes, various toxins are generated that are eliminated by the kidney. Ketosis occurs in type 1 diabetes mellitus due to the absence of insulin, which prevents the use of circulating glucose at the cellular level , as well as in situations of prolonged fasting or after the consumption of so-called ketogenic diets .

It is produced due to excessive accumulation of Acetyl-CoA . In normal state and with sufficient contribution of carbohydrates, these are transformed by the process of glycolysis in pyruvate . Pyruvate by carboxylation causes oxaloacetate , necessary for binding with Acetyl-CoA and entering the citric acid pathway .

The excess of Acetyl-CoA condenses to form acetoacetyl-CoA. The latter compound, through different processes of hydroxylation and hydrolysis , gives rise to acetoacetate, D-3 hydroxybutyrate and acetone: the so-called ketone bodies.

The liver does not have the enzymes necessary to metabolize these compounds, so they are released into the bloodstream to be used by different tissues, especially muscle. When the production of ketone bodies exceeds the use, the phenomenon called ketoacidosis occurs.

CAUSES OF KETOSIS

- Concomitant diseases and infections. The need for insulin increases during these periods.
- I forgot my insulin dose.
- Duration of stress

ADVANTAGES OF KETOSIS

Ketosis has many advantages. Providing almost unlimited energy to the body and brain can improve mental and physical performance. It also reduces hunger and makes weight loss easier.

In addition, the transition to ketosis consumes very little carbohydrate and can effectively treat type 2 diabetes. Ketosis has long been used to control epilepsy.

Beyond this, ketosis has shown many possibilities for the treatment of several other conditions, such as acne relief, PCOS correction, and brain tumor treatment.

HOW TO ENTER KETOSIS

ketosis will be far to get into when hormones have Low levels of insulin and fat storage. ketogenic diet is the diet for solving this.

Values above 3 mmol / l are not necessary. That is, no better or worse results will be obtained than level 1.5–3. Higher values can sometimes mean that you are consuming insufficient food ("starvation ketosis"). For type 1 diabetes, these values can be caused by severe insulin insufficiency which requires urgent medical attention.

Normally it is impossible to reach values that exceed 8–10 mmol / l only by consuming a ketogenic diet. This means that something is wrong. The most common cause by far is type 1 diabetes with a severe lack of insulin.

The symptoms are feeling very sick with nausea,

vomiting, abdominal pain and confusion. The end result may be a life-threatening state called ketoacidosis. Obviously, abnormally high levels of ketones require urgent medical attention.

THE RISKS OF KETOSIS

Although ketosis can offer many advantages, we must know that this state is not risk free , but that it is a process with which we cannot live for a long time and that requires control when induced in the human body

At the time of losing a ketogenic diet, it does not achieve true adherence or what is the same, it is not sustainable in the long term due in large part to the fact that a strict diet is required to sustain this state of ketosis over time.

On the other hand, poorly controlled ketogenic diet or a ketosis that occurs without being induced can lead to electrolyte imbalances and severe dehydration , which if left untreated is also fatal as in the case of those suffering from ketoacidosis as reported in the 2006 before the Atkins diet .

Among other minor side effects, there may be a fall in cognitive performance as noted by American scientists , a situation that can be reversed as the state of ketosis is prolonged.

You can also experience dizziness, bad breath, nausea, constipation, fatigue, cramping (especially when using TCM or medium chain triglycerides), headaches , among other minor consequences.

This has to be a diet to take you to a state of ketosis

To reach a state of ketosis or to form ketone bodies, the restriction of carbohydrates is a requirement , that is, we must considerably limit the main source of energy in our body by eliminating both simple sugars and complex hydrates .

Thus in a normal diet hydrates offer between 40 and 60% of the calories of the day, while in a ketogenic diet or keto diet this percentage is reduced to less than 10 each day.

Protein

The rule indicates that you should not exceed 20 grams of hydrates ingested each day for the body to use glycogen stores until they are finished and then begin to oxidize fats only to reach ketosis.

Thus, in a diet that induces ketosis most of the calories are derived from fats : 60-75%, while proteins cover between 25 and 30% of the energy of the day and therefore, hydrates are barely present being able to even offer less than 5% of the calories of the day.

To achieve this, all types of cereals or legumes and derivatives are eradicated from the diet, and the intake of fruits and vegetables is restricted to the maximum .

The diet must eliminate all types of carbohydrates to cause ketosis

The diet is then based on the consumption of foods high in fat and protein such as meat, eggs, dairy, fish, seafood, nuts, seeds, butter and vegetable oils .

For the aforementioned, the ketogenic diet or necessary to enter ketosis is a limited diet, which requires a lot of control and the elimination of entire food groups in order to reduce hydrates considerably at the daily table. And although it can offer many advantages, it is not free of side effects for the body and health.

SYMPTOMS AND HOW TO KNOW THAT YOU ARE IN KETOSIS

How do you know you are in ketosis? It is possible to measure it by analyzing a urine, blood or breath sample . But there are other signs that indicate it and do not require proof:

Dry mouth and increased thirst : unless you drink enough fluids and consume enough electrolytes, such as salt, you could feel your mouth dry. Try one or two cups of broth daily and as much water as you need.

Increased urine : a certain ketone body,

acetoacetate, can end up in the urine. This allows ketosis to be measured using test strips for urinalysis. Another effect of this may be that you need to go to the bathroom more frequently (at least at the beginning). This is the main cause of increased thirst (see above).

Keto breath: this is because of a ketone body, which is called acetone, and that leaves the body through the breath. 4 It can make your breath smell "fruity," or similar to nail polish remover. This smell also sometimes feels in sweat when a person exercises. Many times it is temporary. Learn more

OTHER LESS SPECIFIC BUT MORE POSITIVE INDICATORS ARE:

Reduced hunger: Many people feel a significant reduction in hunger. 5 This can be caused by an increased ability of the body to feed using its fat deposits. Many people feel great eating only two or three times a day, and end up doing an intermittent form of fasting . It saves time and money, while accelerating weight loss.

An increase in energy : maybe after a few days of feeling tired (the " keto flu ") many people feel a marked increase in their energy levels. It can also be perceived as having a lucid mind, a lack of "brain fog", or even as a feeling of euphoria.

SYMPTOMS OF KETOSIS AND ACIDOSIS

- Incompetence
- stomach ache.
- Nausea or vomiting
- Fruity breath scent.
- Breathing difficulty
- My mouth is dry.
- General collapse

If the situation remains uncorrected, sleep trends and reduced levels of consciousness appear. If evolution continues, you will reach a comma.

KETOSIS AND CANCER

Due to the existence of the Warburg effect , by which cancer cells feed mainly glucose, it is proposed that the presence of glucose in cancers can be key to the development and ketosis and usually keto acids can be beneficial in stopping tumor growth.

It has been observed in several studies in mice, the application of ketogenic diets decreases tumor growth and improves survival in certain laboratory mice with cancer such as brain, colon cancer, gastric cancer and prostate cancer. Other articles indicate that ketogenic diets could function as adjuvants in radiotherapy and cancer chemotherapy. The oxidative stress given in cancer cells would make them more sensitive to these treatments

There are studies that evaluate the possibility of controlling the blood sugar of type 1 and type 2 diabetics through a ketogenic diet. By reducing carbohydrate intake, insulin needs are reduced and glucose levels stabilized.

Ketosis may help treat Alzheimer's disease, according to a study in 152 patients.

When certain diets are followed , such as the Paleolithic diet , the Atkins diet or the Dukan diet , the state of ketosis is promoted based on drastically reducing the intake of carbohydrates . However, in certain forms of epilepsy refractory to usual pharmacological treatments, the use of the ketogenic diet is proposed as a therapeutic alternative.

Although nutritional and medical orthodoxy usually states that the brain "only works with glucose," many studies indicate that ketosis, in addition to not harming the brain, seems to improve its functioning

CHAPTER EIGHT

KETOACIDOSIS

There are many misconceptions about ketosis. The most common mistake is to confuse it with ketoacidosis, an uncommon and dangerous medical condition that occurs mostly to people with type 1 diabetes if they don't take insulin. 6 Even some health care professionals tend to confuse the two situations quite a bit, perhaps due to similar names and a lack of knowledge of the marked differences.

Ketosis and ketoacidosis not are the same.

Ketosis is a completely natural state and under complete control of the body. It can be caused by a ketogenic diet or a short period of fasting.

Ketoacidosis is a serious malfunction of the body where there is an excessive and uncontrolled production of ketones. It generates symptoms such as nausea, vomiting and stomach pains followed by confusion and, finally, going into a coma. It requires urgent medical treatment because it can be deadly. 7

The graph you see below shows the great

difference between blood ketones in case of ketosis and in case of ketoacidosis:

Most people who follow a ketogenic diet never reach higher levels of plus or minus 3 millimolars, and many people have a hard time reaching levels of more than 0.5. Long-term starvation, that is a week or more without food, could cause the figure to rise to 6 or 7. But ketoacidosis occurs at levels of more than 10, and more frequently more than 15.

It is similar to the difference between drinking a glass of water and drowning in the sea. The two situations are about water, but they are not the same. Drinking a glass of water will not make you drown. Similarly, ketosis does not cause ketoacidosis.

If you have a pancreas that works well and can produce insulin, that is, if you don't have type 1 diabetes, it would be very difficult, probably impossible, to have ketoacidosis, even if you tried. The reason is that having high ketone levels causes insulin production, which stops the production of more ketones. In other words, the body has a safety net that normally makes it impossible for healthy people to suffer from ketoacidosis.

WHAT TO EAT ON A KETOGENIC DIET

These are some of the traditional foods that can

be enjoyed with a ketogenic diet. The number is the net carbohydrate per 100 grams. In general, it is better to consume low levels of carbohydrates to maintain ketosis.

The most important thing to achieve ketosis is to avoid eating most carbohydrates. You may need to keep your carbohydrate intake below 50 grams per day and 5 grams below 20 grams. Less carbohydrate are more effective.

TRY TO AVOID

This is something you should not eat on a ketogenic diet. Food filled with sugar and starch, including high starchy foods such as bread, pasta, rice, and potatoes. As you can see, these diets are much higher in carbohydrates.

This means that sweet and starchy foods such as bread, pasta, rice and potatoes must be avoided altogether. Basically, follow strict low-carb diet guidelines and remember to be high fat, not protein.

A rough recommendation is that less than 10% of the energy comes from carbohydrates (the less carbohydrates are more effective), 15-25% of proteins (lower amounts are more effective), and more than 70% fat.

WHAT TO DRINK

So what liquids can you drink on a ketogenic diet?

Drinking water is perfect and coffee, tea and mate are perfect. Do not use sweeteners. A moderate amount of milk, cream, or cream is sufficient (but avoid cappuccino and coffee with milk!) Sometimes you can drink a glass of wine.

KETONE IS BRAIN ENERGY

It is a common misconception that the brain needs carbohydrates. The truth is that when you consume them, the brain burns carbohydrates. However, if you don't eat a lot of carbohydrates, your brain will not have a problem with burning ketones.

This feature is absolutely necessary for basic survival. If this is not the case, the body can only store one or two days of carbohydrate supply, so the brain will immediately fail after a few days without food.

Alternatively, muscle proteins need to be converted to glucose just to maintain brain function-a very inefficient process. This causes atrophy very quickly without food. If so, mankind would not have survived for thousands of years until food was constantly available.

Fortunately, our bodies have evolved to be smarter than this. Normally, fat buildup lasts, so you can survive for weeks or even months without food. Ketosis is a method used by the body to allow the brain to ingest fat deposits.

There is no need to consume any carbohydrates. The brain is happy to eat fat.

Many people feel more energy and mental concentration when their brains have the opportunity to eat ketones made of fat. And of course, if you are trying to lose weight, this will also promote fat burning.

THE BRAIN AND ITS NEED FOR GLYCOGEN

In addition to all this we must point out that the human brain has glucose as its food and therefore when it does not have glucose to feed it does it from ketone bodies. The problem of ketosis is that ketone bodies are acidic, and there are sources that claim that they can only be used by 50% by the brain and the rest must be provided by glucose.

If we take into account this source, by not putting carbohydrates into the body glucose is not produced and therefore it is not fed to the brain as it should and this can suffer some type of degradation, perhaps not very chaotic but if significant that in the long run It can be counterproductive for its proper functioning.

SIDE EFFECTS FEARS AND POSSIBLE DANGERS

During the first week of following a Ketogenic diet

and entering ketosis it is common to experience some side effects. You may suffer from headaches, tiredness, irritability, leg cramps , constipation and heart palpitations .

These side effects are usually relatively mild and temporary, and most of them can be avoided by consuming enough fluids and salt .

SIDE EFFECTS INCLUDES

Dizziness and headaches: this effect passes from the third day, it is the worst, the body has no energy and even if you get up quickly you can get dizzy. The brain needs glycogen (or ketone bodies) to function from there this effect.

Bad breath: when our body has an excess of ketone body these are released through the breath, hence it is recommended to drink plenty of water, there are even people who have presented a metallic taste in their mouth.

Urine with a very strong smell: ketone bodies are also eliminated in the urine so the smell of it becomes stronger.

Strong sweat: ketone bodies are also removed by sweat so it is normal for your smell to become unpleasant

Lack of appetite: Proteins and fats are very satisfying, in addition to the fact that they cost much more to be digested than carbohydrates, hence the appetite goes down considerably.

Nausea, vomiting, abdominal pain, respiratory distress and general decay

Loss of calcium: excess protein favors the loss of calcium by the kidney (which has previously been removed from the bones) and osteoporosis can be favored.

Possible arrhythmias: they may cause problems with the cardiac electrical conduction system and arrhythmias.

Loss of muscle: if it is a long time in ketosis, the fat is pulled first but when it is going down, the muscle begins to degrade to use its amino acids as fuel

The brain and its need for glycogen

In addition to all this we must point out that the human brain has glucose as its food and therefore when it does not have glucose to feed it does it from ketone bodies. The problem with ketosis is that ketone bodies are acidic, and there are sources that claim that they can only be used by 50% by the brain and the rest must be supplied by glucose.

HOW TO REACH KETOSIS

There are many elements that increase the level of ketosis. We detail them below, from the most important to the least important:

Restrict carbohydrate intake to 20 grams digestible or less per day: a strict low carb diet. It is not necessary to restrict fiber consumption, rather it could be beneficial. 12

Restrict protein intake to moderate levels. If possible, keep your protein intake below 1 gram per day for every kg of body weight. So it would be about 70 grams of protein per day if you weigh 70 kilograms (154 pounds). It may be beneficial to lower protein consumption even more, especially if you are overweight, targeting 1 gram of protein per kg of desired weight. The most common mistake, and that prevents people from achieving optimal ketosis, is too high protein intake.

Eat enough fat to feel satisfied. This is the big difference between a ketogenic diet and starvation, which also causes ketosis. A ketogenic diet is sustainable; starvation no.

Avoid snacks when you're not hungry. Unnecessary snacks delay weight loss and reduce ketosis.

If necessary, add a form of intermittent fasting , such as 16/8. This is very effective for stimulating ketone levels, as well as for accelerating weight loss and reversing type 2 diabetes.

Normally not necessary: Supplement the diet with TCM oil (medium chain triglycerides) and / or bulletproof coffee.

Normally not necessary: supplement with exogenous ketones . 13

Two stories about how to achieve optimal ketosis

Below are three reports of a two-month experiment on how to achieve optimal ketosis:

Experiment: optimal ketosis to lose weight and increase physical performance

Four weeks following a strict low carb diet and measuring ketones

Final report: two months of a strict low carb diet and measuring ketones

Do I have to achieve optimal ketosis to experience the benefits?

In short, no. Many of the benefits, such as weight loss, are experienced at lower levels of ketosis (at least above 0.5). There are indications that you might have to reach higher levels of ketosis for high-level physical performance.

HOW IS KETOSIS MEASURED

There are three ways to measure ketones, all have their advantages and disadvantages:

- Urine test strips
- Ketone Breath Analyzers
- Blood ketone meters

CHAPTER NINE

GETTING STARTED MADE EASY

Mechanism of intermittent fasting

Intermittent fasting is not a diet. Intermittent fasting is effective, but diet does not work. Most meals are based on calorie restriction. Instead of eating 1,800 kcal per day, eat 1,200 reduced by 30%. This causes a rapid weight loss, especially for water, muscle mass, and some fats. As soon as you stop dieting, your weight will recover.

Intermittent fasting also means reducing calories, but for a week instead of a day. If the daily meal is 1,800 kcal and you stop eating for two days, the weekly intake will be reduced by 30% after one week. So what is the difference?

The difference is in the adaptability of the body. After a week of starvation on a low-calorie diet, basal metabolism decreases. That means your body spends less than the reduced meal you are already eating. Researchers call this well-known phenomenon "adaptive heat generation", but you will definitely find it as "metabolic damage". That is why the low calorie diet does not work.

The advantage of intermittent fasting is a reduction in calories, but it is not adapted because it fasts for up to 24 hours. You will eat again before your metabolism falls.

In addition, intermittent fasting increases metabolism by up to 14% and maintains it instead of losing muscle.

HOW TO DO IT

While it may not be easy to personally test the effects of intermittent fasting, keep in mind these signs:

The most comfortable way is to get most of the night fasting. For example, you usually eat at noon the day you start, but no longer eat that day. The next day, skip breakfast and have your first meal at noon.

Drink water at high speed as if there was no tomorrow. You can also drink tea, coffee, and generally liquids without calories. No, honey cannot be added to tea.

Start with a fast one day a week. If acclimatization is smooth, it can be done in two consecutive days, such as Tuesday and Friday.

Make sure that your exercise program is closed on the day you start fasting. The next day, exercise just before the first meal.

Avoid prolonged exercise during fasting. When exercising strength or intervals, take a small dose of an amino acid tablet containing protein, shake, or leucine to avoid burning muscle mass.

What happens to you when you are training on an empty stomach?

Studies show that:

You keep the glucose level stable for at least 2 hours of training

You also keep basal insulin levels stable, without fluctuations

The plasma level of fatty acids gradually increases, especially after one hour of exercise.

You use fat as the main energy source and thus the use of glycogen is prevented.

Use intramuscular fatty acids more efficiently

You save glycogen deposits so you can use them in the final stretch of the race, where you have to increase the intensity and win the competition!

You recover more easily, as long as you do it correctly.

You will see an improvement in training performance with 60-70% VO2max intensity

At the level of recovery: it is essential that you follow the advice we have given you in the post about post-exercise feeding. If shortly: after fasting training it is even more important that you consume an adequate amount of carbohydrates and proteins in the anabolic window, because this type of training can cause more damage to proteins, because the body can use protein from the muscles as a source of energy, but with the consumption of protein after exercise the muscle recovers faster. And a good portion of carbohydrates decreases muscle catabolism.

The key to fasting training is light intensity, nothing intensive!

What happens that your body gradually gets used to perceive glycogen as the most valuable thing and spends it only in extreme conditions, and in other periods it spends fat. So when you have competition or a test of intensity higher than training, your body, as I learned in fasting training, will use fat and carbohydrates more effectively. It will not spend all the glycogen at once, but it will spend fat first, and glycogen will save for the final straight. And of course before the competition you have to consume carbohydrates and start the test well hydrated (as always, that never changes) and with glycogen-filled deposits, as we explained in previous posts.

HOW TO FAIL WITH INTERMITTENT FASTING

If you use it to offend you: After the first day of fasting, there are people who take revenge and throw themselves into junk food during the rest of the day. In studies with mice, after fasting, they placed themselves on top and canceled all the beneficial effects. You can fall to the same. Intermittent fasting works only when there is a reduction in total energy, which is achieved by eating the remaining time of protein, vegetables, and control carbohydrates normally. Eating donuts with more than a dozen people is no excuse.

If you don't play sports: Caloric restriction always causes muscle loss, and the best way to avoid it is strength training. Long jogging races are a bad idea because your body can begin to burn muscle mass instead of fat. It is best to do a high intensity exercise or a short session of weight just before the first meal after fasting.

If not intermittent: fasting over 48 hours, sometimes disguised as "cleaning" such as maple syrup diet, onion diet, starving, losing muscle mass, reducing metabolism, you eating again As soon as possible. please do not.

THE GOLDEN KEY OF AUTOPHAGY AND WHY IT IS SO IMPORTANT FOR WOMEN

Fasting rejuvenates our cells by autophagy

It has been known recently that our cells are able to regenerate their damaged or worn out parts over time. Our whole body can benefit from this "cellular rejuvenation".

This process is activated by fasting, even short, but also with other simple methods.

Autophagy: regeneration in our cells

Literally, this word means that our cells "eat themselves". In fact, they dislocate in them worn or foreign particles (thanks to enzymes) to use them eventually later. In some cases, they can "do something new with old" and recycle degraded protein into new cellular components. They can also draw energy from it, as we will see.

This function exists in each of our cells. In fact, this process of cleaning and repair occurs naturally, cyclically, during the phases when the cell is in relative rest, but it tends to become less active with advancing age .

Autophagy of foreign bodies in the disease

Autophagy (or autolysis) allows cells to remove unwanted particles or substances that have been able to enter cells: viruses, bacteria, toxins, degenerate proteins. Thus, it is implicated in infectious diseases but also in neurodegenerative disorders, cancer, etc ... It improves our immune system, reduces inflammation and protects our cardiovascular system, among many other beneficial effects.

AUTOPHAGY WITHOUT DISEASE: A REAL CELL REJUVENATION

Every day, of the millions of reactions that occur in our cells, some have "misfires" and produce abnormal or overused components. During the autophagy of these deteriorated components, a kind of "recycling of defective parts" of the cell is done. These components can be classified among our famous toxins which, over time, "foul" our body.

Autophagy is also described as an alternative source of energy for the cell, implemented during certain stresses such as fasting, low blood sugar, intense efforts, or lack of oxygen ... Clearly, during these periods of stress, the cell generates energy by "burning" its waste.

Your cells can repair themselves cell repair tools

Among the important components of the cell, you may have heard of mitochondria , these "small boilers" that burn oxygen and nutrients to produce your body's energy.

Being the seat of strong oxidizing reactions, their malfunction or deterioration is very detrimental to our health. In fact, free radicals * can then be produced in excess and in turn damage other elements of the cell, even its DNA (which contains our genes) and then leave the cell to attack other tissues.

These oxidation reactions continue until our antioxidant system neutralizes them. Studies have shown correlations between this phenomenon and acceleration of aging, cancer and degenerative diseases.

Thus, autophagy can appear as the anti-aging system of our body . That said, let's not forget that this is a normal phenomenon like other mechanisms of defense and repair of our body and not a miracle cure. The real discovery is that autophagy tends to reduce with age and especially with our poor lifestyle, thus allowing degenerative diseases to settle. The good news is that you can take action to wake up and use this fabulous tool.

AUTOPHAGY AND DEGENERATIVE DISEASES

Studies of neurodegenerative diseases have shown that neurons can eliminate their toxins and regenerate their damaged mitochondria through autophagy. This can be triggered in the brain during a fast and would be much more effective for this than other restrictive diets. This autolysis process can attack the intracellular deposits that occur with aging, especially in diseases such as Alzheimer's.

It has also been shown that activation of autophagy can improve the condition of kidneys damaged by diabetes and may also play a role in osteoarthritis in mice.

Fasting against aging through autophagy

Fasting to rejuvenate?

Fasting promotes autophagy phenomena that allow cellular regeneration and avoid accelerating aging and certain oxidation phenomena. Fasting can be considered as an anti-aging technique.

Rejuvenating has been a human concern for a very long time. "rejuvenation enzyme" and quotes the research on autophagy of Professor Mizushima of Tokyo. He advocates, for his part, mini-fasts from 16 to 24 h, repeated regularly. It is also based on the studies of Pr Panda (La Jolla California) who showed the following:

Mice eating a very high fat and high calorie food, at any time of the day, for 100 days, see their health parameters deteriorate (obesity, excess of fats and sugars in the blood, liver problems).

On the other hand, mice that eat exactly the same thing, in the same quantity but for only 8 hours of the day and fasting during the other 16 hours, do not have these troubles and even see their shape improve. A priori, the metabolism of the body is positively modified by brief periods of fasting (at least for mice).

This seems interesting, especially since Professor Malene Hansen has shown that periods of fasting, inducing autophagy in the worm, could extend its life by 25%! Note however that it is (as often) studies of animals.

Other research goes in this direction. Biologist Pr Ohsumi has dedicated his life to studying the mechanisms of this phenomenon (Nobel Prize 2016) and its implications in the fight against degenerative diseases, cancer, infections.

Finally, it seems that most of the techniques that have succeeded in lengthening life expectancy in experimental models of genetic manipulation or the administration of substances (such as resveratrol, lithium, rapamycin ...), finally stimulate autophagy.

This cellular process seems very interesting to rejuvenate a body in its entirety and to maintain health. In addition, its effects would be particularly convincing in the skin.

FASTING AND TRADITIONS

It can be noted that, often, the populations rich in centenarians know periods of scarcity where they do not necessarily eat every day or at every meal. Would that contribute to their steel health and longevity? It's possible.

Most religions require periods of food restriction or fasting. It is usually a day of fasting weekly or alternative fasting as in Ramadan where it is allowed to eat at night. If we take away the hours of sleep, we are close to fasting from 16 to 18 hours.

Traditional medicine does not advocate long fasts in the lifestyle. They are used to treat diseases, where they are very effective. On the other hand, she advises a weekly day of fasting, routinely, to release Ama (toxins) and regenerate Agni (our digestive capacity) by putting the stomach at rest.

This day adapts to the constitution of the patient (total fasting or liquid diet or very light). In some cases, it may be to simply remove a meal a day to lighten the digestive and toxin load.

Naturopathy has long taught that during a fast, the body draws intelligently in its reserves, it first draws in fat, then in damaged tissues, then in the less important tissues, etc. Once again science tells us that these concepts were not only imaginary.

TIPS AND TRICKS TO IMPROVE YOUR GENERAL HEALTH

We all want to keep steel healthy and improve the general condition. After looking for formulas to know what to do about health for years, I concluded that I could participate in the most important points to consider with 10 tips that should not be missed. I would like to share with you all the experiences that belong to us all. It is to know what we should do to become healthy and healthy.

Sports practice:

Realization of sports, sport is one of the best ways to stay young and perfect as it helps keep your body active and keep your muscles tight and strong. For sports, it is ideal to avoid getting used to the same activities that change, so you need to run at least three sessions a week, regardless of activity. Personally, I believe that diversity is indispensable when playing sports. In addition to not getting tired, your body will always have to face new challenges, so you will get better results.

Respect the rest:

Rest another point that must be taken into account. And it is important that we sleep 7-8 hours a day so that our bodies are in perfect condition. Rest is essential for muscle recovery after training and daily activities. Remember that sleep can also help improve oxygenation and skin condition and improve the overall functioning of all organs of the body.

Maintain a proper diet:

Maintain a diet that must be diverse. Following a diet with different types of food is essential to achieving health. Our bodies are ready to absorb all kinds of food, and all these foods provide us with a set of nutrients necessary to achieve health. Therefore, it is necessary to utilize all kinds of food. The advice I give you is to get a Mediterranean meal as an example. Because it accepts a diverse and balanced diet

Note saturated fat:

Saturated fat and abuse are other tips. Because our bodies need fat to live, it is important to eat fat, but it is important to know what types of fats are appropriate to stay healthy. We need to choose monounsaturated and polyunsaturated fats that help the body make the most of it and maintain its integrity.

Make 5 meals.

Not skipping meals is essential to being in the best shape. Hungry is the worst thing we can do to stay healthy. You need to keep track of your meal time and respect it. It is appropriate to make 5 snacks a day. One piece of advice I give you is to divide it into five meals given the amount of food we consume per day. That means you don't have to eat any more to eat more food. The same, but more distributed to win control hunger and maintain the line.

Eat fruits and vegetables:

The inclusion of fruits and vegetables in the diet is essential to keep us in top condition. Fruit provides the vitamins and minerals necessary for the proper functioning of the body. One point to consider for fruits and vegetables is high fiber content. This will help cleanse the body.

Avoid stress:

Alleviating and avoiding stressful situations every day can help improve our health. I think that activities that can avoid everyday life are necessary. Relaxation sessions, yoga, hobbies, sports ... it is highly recommended that the activities that relax us are in perfect condition.

Avoid alcohol and tobacco:

Needless to say, in addition to accelerating the human body's natural aging process, we need to avoid excess of our lives and evil, such as alcohol and tobacco, which deteriorate health at various levels. Controlling this is essential to maintaining proper health. I recommend simply replacing the tip and weighing what these vices mean at a health level.

Hydrate properly:

It can never be ignored. That is proper hydration. Many of our body compositions are liquid. Because water is indispensable for life, you need to provide the body with the amount you need. Therefore, to maintain the proper health of each organ in our body, it is necessary to drink an average of 2 liters of water a day.

Habit planning and management:

The last important tip is planning and management when maintaining good habits. Set a meal schedule. Set up meal schedules, manage meals and dishes, and be prepared to maintain meal diversity. Also set up training and sports schedules. This simple gesture is one of the best ways to achieve complete goals and have complete control over what you are doing.

THE BEST WAY TO USE INTERMITTENT FASTING FOR MUSCLE GAIN

Normally intermittent fasting is associated with weight loss and it is logical since we are controlling feeding periods or schedules and therefore caloric intake.

However, intermittent fasting can also be used if you are looking to increase your muscle mass and here I will tell you how you can do it.

The key to gaining muscle mass while doing intermittent fasting consists of two important points. The number one point is to consume more calories than your body needs per day, that is, above your basal metabolic rate.

It is not necessary that you consume excess

calories, the point is to consume between 200 and 300 calories above or even at your maintenance level. In this way you will avoid accumulating fat . Therefore, it is important that you know what your maintenance level is so that you do not make mistakes, end up eating too much and accumulate fat.

Of course, if you are doing intermittent fasting, it is harder for you to eat so many calories. For example, suppose you need to consume 2,500 calories or more, if you are fasting for 24 hours it will be very difficult for you to consume all those calories in a meal.

I do not say that it is impossible, many people can eat that and even more, however, some people can find it complicated.

So that it is not so complicated I will give you two tips that can work for you if you are thinking of making a big meal.

First you can make a small meal of about 500 calories a few hours before your main meal. In this way your caloric intake in your main meal will be reduced a little.

And second add natural fats to your food. Do not be afraid of fats, this macronutrient is not the culprit of gaining weight, they are the extra calories no matter what macronutrient group it is.

I advise you to add natural fats because fats are the macronutrient with the highest caloric density. There are 9 calories per gram of fat, unlike proteins and carbohydrates that only have 4 calories per gram. In this way about two tablespoons of olive oil, for example, can give you about 180 or 200 calories more. Use it in your favor.

Now if you are fasting 16: 8 it is easier for you to consume all your calories, since you have an 8 hour window to do it.

If we take the same example of 2,500 calories you can make two meals of 1,250 or even two meals of 1,000 and one of 500.

I remember that by intermittent fasting you will have many benefits such as stimulating adrenaline , growth hormone (which is essential for muscle development) and also you will not be preparing meals or interrupting your day 5 or 6 times to eat.

Remember not to exceed your calories a lot, if you do you can accumulate extra fat, even if you are doing intermittent fasting.

And the second key point you should consider to increase your muscle mass is to increase your strength in the exercise through progressive overload.

The progressive overload is to gradually increase

the weight you lift in your gym sessions. It doesn't matter if it's the smallest disk, the goal is to increase your strength little by little.

My recommendation (is what I do) is that you go to the gym 3 days a week on non-consecutive days, that is, Monday, Wednesday and Friday.

In this way you give the body time to recover between each session and therefore you will be able to lift more and more weight.

I also recommend that you keep a record of the weights you are lifting in each exercise so that in this way you carry a tighter control.

Remember that you have to learn to listen to your body, do not overdo it and increase the weights a lot since you can hurt yourself. Try to go slowly and be constant.

And finally as a summary remember to consume about 200 or 300 calories above your maintenance level and increase your strength in your gym sessions through progressive overload. Be constant both in food and exercise.

COMMON MISTAKES WHILE FASTING AND HOW TO AVOID THEM

Fasting under a certain pattern can help us when it comes to losing weight. It is something of which there is evidence. To take advantage of its benefits we can use several nutritional strategies. One of the most efficient is intermittent fasting, a relatively simple pattern to implement in our day to day.

But all that glitters is not gold. We cannot launch to practice it without taking into account some things. Begin intermittent fasting without a little preparation; planning is a safe bet to make a mistake. A mistake that could cost us our entire strategy, today we talk about some of these, to be able to circumvent them effectively.

Intermittent fasting, what can go wrong?

The moment of truth arrives, it is time to move on to intermittent fasting. You are aware that it is not a magic measure, that it will not solve all your problems and that it will not have effects if you do not strain. With all that in mind, what can go wrong? Many things:

Begin intermittent fasting without preparation

Fasting is not easy, no matter how much you think so. You can get it for a while. But if you do not carry a certain preparation, the safest thing is that you do not spend the first few weeks. The fault is not only of your mind, but also of your body . It is necessary to adapt our metabolism to fasting periods. In fact, this justifies, in part, some of its benefits.

Adapting to fasting is something progressive,

which can be done by spacing meals and times between them, reducing the amounts of intake, etc. We can begin to adopt the fast progressively, until we do it on a regular basis. If we throw ourselves in the head, there is a good chance we will lose the battle. But there is still more to this war.

Fasting too long

Like the previous mistake, and for the same reasons, the longer the fast, the harder it will be to maintain it. "If I start doing something, I start it well." This is a mistake. Not to make the fasting longer is more positive nor will we get more benefits. The benefits of fasting are noticed from leaving about 12 hours between intakes, and depend more on the rest of the diet than on the hours themselves. It is better to make fasts more affordable but bearable, than to make them longer and break them shortly.

Think too much about fasting

The mental factor is important. In addition to our metabolism, our head must be in tune to be able to deal with it properly. Therefore, it is not enough just to prepare physically, but also mentally. And how? Stop thinking about fasting better to make a mistake than to maintain an obsessive attitude with fasting

To think about it too much (when we are going to

eat, that if we have to start at such an hour, that if how much time is left ...) it is a safe way to not be able to cope with it. Is there a better strategy? Yes, of course: entertain us. Continuing with our normal life and taking advantage of the most delicate moments to entertain ourselves with something particular (a book, a game, a hobby) is a fairly intelligent method to engage in fasting.

Do not plan your fast

Fast

Planning is the best of your allies in nutritional matters. It can be a bit annoying in the first instance, but it's all about customs. What type of fast are you going to do, the one of 16/8, the one of 24 or the one of 48? What will you eat when you are not fasting? Are you going to do it alone? Had you had that dinner tomorrow night? Can you fast at work? If you do not plan your strategy properly, it is very possible that you take a false step and have a hard time keeping up.

Have high expectations in your fasting plan

Fasting can be a considerable effort and, therefore, you may expect a reward accordingly. Do not put all the meat on the grill. Fasting is not a panacea. Nor is it in itself a solution. Actually, it serves as a booster, an enhancer; of a healthy diet as it helps adjust our metabolism to circadian rhythms. This can improve caloric expenditure and fat metabolism, enhancing weight loss. But we cannot think that it is a magical effect, nor that it has a sensitive effect. It is a phenomenon that will help in the long term, as part of a larger metabolic set.

Not hold on long enough

Like waiting too long, it's also easy to wait too soon. As we have already said, fasting helps to enhance a much broader metabolic set. It is impossible for us to notice the effects quickly. That, sometimes, is confused and makes us give up on our efforts . In order not to fall into error, it is best not to wait too long, not to become obsessed with the results and move forward, planning, for an elongated time, how much time are we talking about? According to the studies, we will see the results with at least one month of intermittent fasting, although we probably need at least three.

Think you can eat whatever you want

One of the most widespread mistakes is to believe that it doesn't matter what you can eat during the hours that you don't have to fast. This is a big mistake. Intermittent fasting is completely useless if we do not raise it with maturity, seeking the necessary caloric deficit. It is useless to fast 12 or 20 hours if in the other 12 or four we put between kilos of sugar and fat between our chest and back.

Intermittent fasting is a measure, as we explained,

to enhance the effects of a healthy diet, not to replace them (which make no sense). If we also add some exercise, or an increase in physical activity, we will see that the benefits of intermittent fasting are even greater.

CHAPTER TEN

KETO DIET AND INTERMITTENT FASTING

One completely changes what you eat (Keto diet includes eating healthy fats that are almost free of protein and carbohydrates), and the other changes when you eat (intermittent) A typical fast does not eat 16 hours a day, but you want 8 you can eat anything).

But there is one thing in common. This is ketosis

the state where the body begins to burn fat for energy, not carbohydrates, can be achieved in two ways.

It makes sense that sometimes they are related, but if you follow them at the same time, can you burn fatter, or it is a more limited practice than just following a Ketogenic diet

Why do you fast on a keto diet

Intermittent fasting can contribute to the keto diet combustion process, some people (including them) use intermittent fasting to initiate ketosis. Intermittent fasting can lower blood sugar levels, which can increase or increase ketosis when ketosis is no longer followed, for example, when you stop dieting.

Keep in mind that it is difficult to follow a keto diet, but it is even more difficult to do intermittent fasting in combination with this diet. Combining those works well with your pace of life and it is not sustainable unless you can commit.

Should I do an intermittent fast on a keto diet

It is not necessary, but not impossible, to intermittently fast the keto diet (mainly because it does not limit caloric intake during the period you can eat).

Roehl believes that the frequency of fasting intermittently is higher than expected. Did you eat dinner at 8pm but did not eat or drink until noon the next day? Well, it's an intermittent fast.

However, if you are using insulin in diabetes, or if you are on a keto diet for any medical reasons such as epilepsy, do not fast intermittently under any circumstances (or actually follow the keto diet) Don't)

What else do I need to know before trying to fast intermittently on the keto diet

Pay close attention to the proportion of ketosis (as a reminder, these are 60-75% calories from fat, 15-30% calories from protein, and 5-10% calories from carbohydrates).

Next, try to eat enough nutrients (that is, less processed). "Ket diets are often considered bacon and cheese dishes, but these foods require less specific nutrients to improve health,"

Intermittent fasting with a keto diet helps burn fat faster and lose weight, but as always, the healthiest and most sustainable diet is something you can really follow. There are intermittent fasts combined with keto diets that may be difficult to maintain for long periods of time.

INTERMITTENT FASTING - CRITICISM

For many people, the goal of intermittent fasting is to lose weight and lose body fat. Which for many is certainly the right and healthiest way, is not the right and healthiest way for all or pregnant and breastfeeding women, for example, and, for girls with (hypothalamic) amenorrhea

If you are affected by irregular or missed periods, please do not worry about fighting your body fat percentage. A study by the University of Copenhagen shows why. I'll call her:

"The Period Study"

The "period study" is actually called "Within-day energy deficiency and reproductive function in female endurance athletes" and was published in November 2017 by the University of Copenhagen.

The Scandinavian research team presented the results of a study of 25 professional endurance athletes, 10 of whom had normal periods and 15 were affected by "menstrual dysfunctions" (symptoms such as irregular or missed periods). 11 of the 15 girls had amenorrhea.

The exciting thing about the situation was that the athletes had almost no differences in age, height, weight or BMI. The girls were on average 26.6 years old, 1.70m tall and had a BMI of 20.6.

But there was an obvious difference: some had their periods, others did not. What was different? Two points are striking:

INTERMITTENT FASTING MYTHS

INTERMITTENT FASTING SLOWS DOWN YOUR METABOLISM AND PUTS YOUR BODY IN "STARVATION MODE

Very curiously, there are studies that show that at least until day 3 of a complete fast , the metabolism increases ; does not decrease :

Resting energy expenditure in short-term starvation is increased as a result of an increase in serum norepinephrine. The cardiovascular, metabolic and hormonal changes accompanying acute starvation in men and women

Enhanced thermogenic response to epinephrine after 48-h starvation in humans

From the third day of fasting, however, it is possible that the metabolism decreases (which makes all the evolutionary sense of the world): Leucine, glucose, and energy metabolism after 3 days of fasting in healthy human subjects

But since it is very characteristic of science, many times things are not only white or black: the following study did observe a reduction in metabolism in conditions more similar to those in the real world:

INTERMITTENT FASTING DOES NOT AFFECT WHOLE-BODY GLUCOSE, LIPID, OR PROTEIN METABOLISM

While the following study found no difference in metabolism after 3 weeks of intermittent fasting, even after participants lost weight (which would be expected, since losing weight does reduce, without any discussion, basal metabolism) :

Alternate-day fasting in nonobese subjects: effects on body weight, body composition, and energy metabolism

Do not waste a second worrying about a reduction in your metabolism. In the event that your metabolism decreases, the effect would be virtually the same as you would experience with any other eating pattern (and more specifically, with any hypocaloric diet). (And no: your body will not go into "starvation mode" or make you accumulate a lot of calories and fat) .

There are many people who have achieved fantastic results by intermittent fasting, and their metabolisms are perfectly normal

INTERMITTENT FASTING MAKES YOU LOSE A LOT OF MUSCLE

It is true that most studies suggest that intermittent fasting is not ideal for building muscle. But this does not mean (not far away) that suddenly you will lose all your muscle mass by spending a few hours without eating.

You have for example the following study, where

intermittent fasting, consuming all calories in a window of 8 hours a day (fasting 16/8), was just as effective as a normal diet to maintain muscle mass during the 2 months that The experiment lasted:

Effects of eight weeks of time-restricted feeding (16/8) on basal metabolism, maximal strength, body composition, inflammation, and cardiovascular risk factors in resistance-trained males

And as in the previous case: many people have built a lot of muscle by intermittent fasting.

FUN FACTS OF INTERMITTENT FASTING

1. The longest fast in history lasted 382 days. Yes … more than a year of fasting living basically based on water and supplements. It was the case of a 27-year-old boy who suffered from obesity and who lost up to 125 kg in the process.

2. Not all studies of intermittent fasting in animals show that fasting extends life; some show that shortens. Effects of intermittent feeding upon body weight and lifespan in inbred mice: interaction of genotype and age

Or of this one, much more interesting, where 41 mouse subspecies were analyzed and it was found that intermittent fasting shortened life in most subspecies and only extended it in the minority:

Genetic variation in the murine lifespan response to dietary restriction: from life extension to life shortening

3. In healthy people, 24 hours of fasting decreases glycogen stores up to 57% .

The effects of fasting and re-feeding with a 'metabolic preconditioning' drink on substrate reserves and mononuclear cell mitochondrial function. As a detail, this study instructed participants to remain at rest during the fasting period, so if you do physical activity (for example), the values would obviously change.

But it is curious to see how the liver is able to continue giving energy to the body even after 24 hours of fasting.

DISADVANTAGES OF INTERMITTENT FASTING

Unlike other diets and eating patterns, intermittent fasting has no significant negative effects (as long as it is not taken to the extreme). Fasting is nothing new to man and would not make much evolutionary sense that would pose a serious threat to his health.

However, minor negative effects such as:

- Fatigue
- Weakness
- Dizziness

- Headache
- Lack of concentration
- Sickness
- Sleep disturbance

The effects of intermittent or continuous energy restriction on weight loss and metabolic disease risk markers: a randomized trial in young overweight women. But these disadvantages are rather temporary while the body adapts to the new eating pattern.

A major disadvantage for those who exercise may be the limitation of increased muscle mass, sports performance, or maximum strength. Here the studies are mixed, but generally they point out that intermittent fasting is not the best way to optimize this type of objectives.

A final negative aspect may be the inappropriate consumption of nutrients: by limiting the hours of food (or the number of meals itself), it is possible to consume less food, and consuming less food, fewer nutrients are consumed.

There are two disadvantages that are not directly caused by intermittent fasting itself, but that are related to it:

- Sustainability.
- Greater attention to food and possible stress.

These "disadvantages" are rather subjective and

dependent aspects of each person (if you have trouble implementing or maintaining intermittent fasting or spend all day thinking about food and that causes you stress, the problem may not be fasting itself, but to you, particularly, it doesn't work for you).

RECOMMENDATIONS FOR INTERMITTENT FASTING

Do you want to try intermittent fasting

Then follow these recommendations so that everything goes smoothly:

1. Take care of your hydration

The lack of food and / or drinks during fasting can cause a slight state of dehydration.

Therefore, be sure to drink at least enough water to maintain adequate levels of hydration. This can also help you prevent undesirable effects such as headache or lack of concentration.

2. Take care of your diet

As you saw in the "Disadvantages of Intermittent Fasting" section, intermittent fasting can compromise the intake of important nutrients by reducing meal times or the number of meals themselves.

To ensure an adequate supply of nutrients to your body, choose nutritious foods (as you should do in any diet) and start your meals with those foods (if you leave them for the end, you could end up too full and not consume the nutrients you need) .

Also, consider varying your options and not eating the same foods over and over again (with a little enough; not much variation is necessary).

3. Fast Strategically

Fast at least it costs you.

It could be, for example, when you are very busy with your work or very focused on a particular task or activity. That will help you make fasting more bearable and avoid excessive attention in food. Also consider fasting when your physical activity is low.

If you match your fast with periods of high physical activity, the combination of low calorie availability with high caloric expenditure can not only decrease your energy and make you feel physically and emotionally bad, but compromise your ability to adapt and recover and, at In the long run, do not get the best results.

4. Remember that Calories Keep Counting

Do not fall into the error of thinking that by skipping one or two meals, you can eat everything in sight and still lose weight.

Fasting can help control calories, but if you are not careful, it is not difficult (at all) to pass. You consume your calories in 24, 12, 8, 4 or even 2 hours, what will make you lose weight is how many calories you consume; Not when you consume them.

5. Concentrate Meals Around Exercise

Doing so will help you have (and put) more energy into your workouts and recover better, so you could achieve better long-term results. For example, if you decide to make 3 meals during your feeding period, you can make one meal before your workout and the other two after.

You could also try to decrease your calories and / or make a longer fast on your rest days and increase them and / or make a shorter fast on your training days.

Finally (and especially if your goal is to increase muscle mass), consider consuming protein in a distributed way (do not make a single meal a day, for example).

6. Give your body time to adapt

As usually happens when the body undergoes major changes, the process of adaptation to intermittent fasting can take time. But if after that time, your mind and body do not feel at ease with the new eating pattern, intermittent fasting may not be for you.

7. Take it Calm

In the "Disadvantages of Intermittent Fasting" section, you saw that intermittent fasting has no serious negative health effects. But do you know something that makes health much worse?

Stress .

If intermittent fasting causes you stress, it will have far more important repercussions for you than any positive effect that fasting can bring you .

If you are fasting 16/8 (for example) and when it has been 15 hours you get hungry and you start to ask yourself "Can I eat that apple? What happens if I break my fast? Will I throw everything overboard? "... Look at it as a sign that you may be taking it too seriously.

Relax, it's not that serious .

Your body is very intelligent and will not change its machinery dramatically because you spend a few more hours or a few hours less without eating.

One last piece of advice I could give you is that the types of intermittent fasting are nothing more than standard and common models that people use and are used in scientific studies.

But is it really necessary that you follow them to the letter?

Do not.

Start small, experiment with different durations of fasting and food, move your stripes at different times of the day, try to eat something small if you cannot spend many hours without eating.

Find a model you like, you work, and you feel good to you.

If you like the idea and have the time, consider doing cardio during your fast . For many people, the combination of fasting with exercise makes them feel very good mentally and mentally.

If you feel "off", very low energy or even start to get dizzy during exercise, lower the intensity and / or duration, and if necessary, consider going home . Your body will adapt as you practice intermittent fasting more, but if during the adaptation process you experience some of these symptoms, take it as a sign that it was perhaps too much for your body.

FREQUENTLY ASKED QUESTIONS

WHAT IS FASTING

Fasting is defined as the act of totally or partially abstaining from eating or drinking for a period of time, this may be voluntary or imposed. Perhaps you have heard that in most religions some form of fasting is practiced, it may be a special day a week or at certain times of the year. Apart from the religious, today many people fast in a complementary way to detox processes.

IS FASTING AND DETOX THE SAME

Although the public generally relates to fasting with detox or purification, and while they are practices that are related, as you can review here , they are not the same. A detox can be performed without having to fast because one of the objectives is to facilitate the disposal of waste products such as heavy metals. On the other hand, fasting, depending on the type of fasting, has different objectives, usually what is sought is to optimize our metabolism and reconnect with the signals of our body.

WHAT DO YOU MEAN BY "TYPES OF FASTING"

First of all, you need to know that there are 2 major types of fasting:

Intermittent fasting: refers to periods of fasting during the same day or for several days a week. It is a practice that can be done on a regular basis.

Long fasting: refers to fasting periods of several days, more than 3 days and up to 40 days, may be accompanied by green juices or only with water. It is a practice that should be advised and is recommended a few times a year.

CAN FASTING BE PRACTICED AS A LIFESTYLE

Yes you can, and that is the idea! In this case, intermittent fasting is recommended. We discuss the variants of this type of fasting:

5: 2 This type of intermittent fasting is a practice in which it is recommended to eat without restrictions for 5 days a week and intercalated, every 2 days, consume with a calorie restriction at 500Kcal per day. Example: normal Monday and Tuesday, Wednesday fast, Thursday and normal Friday, Saturday fast, etc.

8 hours to eat: These types of intermittent fasting recommend a continuous fast for at least 16 hours and consume all the food you need daily in a time window of 8 hours. Example: You fast from 8 pm and eat after noon.

Other variants: we can also find different formats that combine these types of intermittent fasting, for example: some of them are "protocols" with fewer fasting hours per day or having more fasting days per week

HOW DO YOU DIET WHEN FASTING

Eat Stop Eat fasting diet

Eat normally for 5 days, then fast for 24 hours twice per week.

During normal eating days, eat nutritious foods, but do not eliminate food groups or give up the foods you love — your fasting time provides all the calorie restriction you need.

HOW MUCH WEIGHT YOU CAN LOSE IN A MONTH WITH INTERMITTENT FASTING

Intermittent fasting weight loss studies are usually investigating fasting interventions every other day, lasting 5: 2 meals or 3-6 months. For most people in such studies, it takes 2-3 months to lose 10 pounds.

HOW LONG SHOULD I TAKE TO SEE THE RESULTS OF INTERMITTENT FASTING

After a week, sugar cravings will be reduced, bowel movements will be regular, and weight loss results will vary, but AEN peep will lose 1-5 pounds in the first week of a 21-day intermittent fasting program.

INTERMITTENT FASTING IS DANGEROUS

Intermittent fasting increases cortisol levels and makes you feel stressed. Early studies found that intermittent fasting could reduce the risk of diabetes, cancer, and heart disease.

CAN I DRINK FLUIDS DURING FASTING

Yes. Water, coffee or tea and other non-caloric drinks. Do not add sugar to coffee and keep in mind that small amounts of milk or cream are also a good option. Coffee can be especially beneficial during fasting, as it helps to kill hunger.

IS IT HEALTHY TO SKIP BREAKFAST

No. The problem is that people who usually skip breakfast have unhealthy lifestyles. If you make sure you eat healthy foods for the rest of the day, fasting is perfectly healthy.

CAN I TAKE SUPPLEMENTS WHILE FASTING

Yes. However, keep in mind that some supplements such as fat-soluble vitamins may work better if they are accompanied with meals.

CAN I EXERCISE WHILE FASTING

Yes of course. Some people recommend taking branched-chain amino acids (BCAA) before exercising.

DOES FASTING CAUSE MUSCLE LOSS

All methods of losing weight can cause muscle loss, so it is important to lift weights and maintain a high protein intake. One study showed that intermittent fasting causes much less muscle loss than a normal calorie restriction.

CAN FASTING SLOW MY METABOLISM

No. Studies show that short-term fasts raise the metabolism. However, if they are performed in the long term for 3 or more days it can inhibit the metabolism.

CAN FASTING BE DANGEROUS

Fasting is not without risks

Fasting cures should improve health, but if misused, there are some risks that, in the worst-case scenario, can affect or even harm your health. The typical risks include muscle breakdown or acidity of the body.

WHAT CAN I EAT WHILE FASTING

Refrain from eating for a week, drinking only tea, water, juices and vegetable broth - and still experiencing unforeseen forces, intoxicating feelings of happiness and losing a few pounds. This is what fasting people promote

WHAT CAN ONE DRINK AT INTERVAL FASTING

You must pay attention to this during interval fasting

In both variants it is important not to eat more than usual in the phases of food intake. You can and should drink while fasting - but only calorie-free drinks such as water, thin vegetable broth, unsweetened tea or moderately black coffee.

WHAT IS FASTING GOOD FOR

Why fasting is good. Fasting can have a healing effect on some illnesses, but fasting is also a way for healthy people to do something good for the body. A fasting cure can take place throughout the year - regardless of the Christian Lent between Ash Wednesday and Easter.

IS COFFEE ALLOWED AT INTERVAL FASTING

Generally speaking, nothing against coffee at Intervals fast. The coffee should only be drunk without milk and without sugar. This cappuccino, latte macchiato and milk coffee are unfortunately taboo. Coffee not only cheerfully but also serves as an appetite suppressant and can even have an analgesic effect.

HOW LONG CAN YOU FAST WITHOUT EATING SOMETHING

The period without solid food should last at least ten days, but not more than five weeks. Thereafter, the energy reserves of the body are consumed and it may be deficiency symptoms. Fasting is especially difficult during the first two to four days.

WHAT ARE NUTRIWHITE'S INDICATIONS FOR INTERMITTENT FASTING

A: We believe that most people can practice intermittent fasting every day. It can become a lifestyle , with the following recommendations: Your fast should start at night with dinner (overnight fasting) and last between 14 and 16 hours to get the benefits.

However, you must start small. If you normally do 8 hours of fasting, try to do 9 hours and so on until you reach the goal. Otherwise it will be counterproductive. It's like wanting to run a marathon, and never having practiced for it.

You don't need to "skip" any food, just adjust the times when you are going to eat.

It is useless to perform this practice if at the end of the fast your diet is based on processed and / or pro-inflammatory foods.

Listen to your body, fasting is to benefit you, not to make you feel bad, so it is vital that you evaluate the tolerance of your own organism.

IS THE PRACTICE OF FASTING FOR EVERYONE

A: Any health recommendation should be as

individualized as possible . Not everyone tolerates the same foods; not everyone has the same physical capacity; some suffer from diabetes, others from arthritis; some people want to lose weight; Others gain muscle mass. In the same way, practicing a fast in a way that is therapeutic will depend on the person's tolerance and goals.

According to the American Academy of Nutrition and Dietetics, a very long fast is not appropriate for pregnant women, children, people with diabetes, especially those who are insulin dependent and people who take special medications. In this case, shorter fasts of 10 to 12 hours are recommended.

DOES INTERMITTENT FASTING CAUSE KETOSIS

In blood samples, those who fasted for 12-24 hours had a 60% increase in energy from fat, with the greatest change occurring after 18 hours. This is an advantage of intermittent fasting because it is called a "ketosis "not necessarily fasting to increase ketone levels

CONCLUSION

In conclusion, fasting is a super powerful tool to improve health but should be used wisely and gradually. I want to finish this article with the following tips.

- Do not use intermittent fasting with the mentality of losing weight but of improving your health. Weight loss will come by itself when your body is ready to release fat.
- Never do intermittent fasting in conjunction with the ketogenic diet or any other diet unless you have already practiced the diet for some time and your body is accustomed to that style of eating. It is better to start with the ketogenic diet and then add intermittent fasting as an extra tool to boost your metabolism.
- Always listen to your body! Never force him to fast more than he can tolerate.

Intermittent fasting is a simple diet in which we use a prolonged fast of 16 hours or more with the aim of achieving better weight control, improve cardiovascular health, decrease the incidence of neurodegenerative diseases, control the systemic inflammation, and improve insulin sensitivity and other metabolic problems.

There is a protocol of 16 hours and one of 24 hours which we can perform on a daily, inter-daily, or weekly basis, depending on the circumstances.

It is recommended to gradually increase fasting periods and always listen to our body. It does not have to be a restrictive regime and will gradually be associated with the reduction of hunger and a greater sense of satiety.

It is a powerful tool, not only for weight control, but to improve our cardiovascular and metabolic health. It is a way of spacing feeding schedules to multiply the benefits of a healthy diet and prevent multiple diseases and health problems.

Intermittent fasting has its pros and cons. The good thing is that these cons are not so serious if you practice a healthy intermittent fasting. Some people work very well with intermittent fasting; others not.

But since one of the main reasons why many decide to intermittent fasting is to lose weight and / or improve their health, do not forget that: Intermittent fasting may be an effective strategy to lose weight, but it is not superior to daily / continuous caloric restriction.

As with any diet (be it Ketogenic, Paleolithic, vegan), intermittent fasting will help you lose weight only if you maintain a caloric deficit for long enough. If you go over calories, you will gain weight (and that can happen with or without fasting).

Although much remains to be studied, the benefits of intermittent fasting in terms of health are similar to those that any other diet that is also healthy can provide.

Finally, follow these intermittent fasting tips

- Fast two or three times a week, but on non-consecutive days.
- On fasting days do yoga, stretching or light cardio.
- Ideally, fast for 12-16 hours.
- Eat normally on those days when you are going to do more intense cardio exercises.
- Consider taking 5-8 grams of BCAAs during fasting days.
- Drink all the water you want. Coffee and tea are also allowed.
- Once you're comfortable with this (more or less after two or three weeks), don't cut yourself into fasting more often and add details like fasting for more hours during weekends and fewer hours during the week.

www.ingramcontent.com/pod-product-compliance
Lightning Source LLC
Chambersburg PA
CBHW070835250726
48662CB00003B/1230